Behavioral H[...]

Editors

KIM ZUBER
JANE S. DAVIS

PHYSICIAN ASSISTANT CLINICS

www.physicianassistant.theclinics.com

Consulting Editor
JAMES A. VAN RHEE

July 2021 • Volume 6 • Number 3

ELSEVIER

1600 John F. Kennedy Boulevard • Suite 1800 • Philadelphia, Pennsylvania, 19103-2899

http://www.theclinics.com

PHYSICAL ASSISTANT CLINICS Volume 6, Number 3
July 2021 ISSN 2405-7991, ISBN-13: 978-0-323-79118-2

Editor: Katerina Heidhausen
Developmental Editor: Axell Ivan Jade Purificacion

Physician Assistant Clinics (ISSN: 2405–7991) is published quarterly by Elsevier Inc., 360 Park Avenue South, New York, NY 10010-1710. Months of issue are January, April, July, and October. Periodicals postage paid at New York, NY and additional mailing offices. Subscription prices are $150.00 per year (US individuals), $290.00 (US institutions), $100.00 (US students), $150.00 (Canadian individuals), $297.00 (Canadian institutions), $100.00 (Canadian students), $150.00 (international individuals), $297.00 (international institutions), and $100.00 (international students). Foreign air speed delivery is included in all *Clinics* subscription prices. All prices are subject to change without notice. POSTMASTER: Send address changes to *Physician Assistant Clinics*, Elsevier Periodicals Customer Service, 11830 Westline Industrial Drive, St. Louis, MO 63146. Customer Service Health Sciences Division, Subscription Customer Service, 3251 Riverport Lane, Maryland Heights, MO 63043. **Customer Service: 1-800-654-2452 (U.S. and Canada); 314-447-8871 (outside U.S. and Canada). Fax: 314-447-8029. E-mail: journalscustomerservice-usa@elsevier.com (for print support); journalsonlinesupport-usa@elsevier.com (for online support).**

Reprints. For copies of 100 or more, of articles in this publication, please contact the Commercial Reprints Department, Elsevier Inc., 360 Park Avenue South, New York, NY 10010-1710. Tel. 212-633-3874; Fax: 212-633-3820; E-mail: reprints@elsevier.com.

Physician Assistant Clinics is covered in *EMBASE/Excerpta Medica* and *ESCI*.

PROGRAM OBJECTIVE

The goal of the *Physician Assistant Clinics* is to keep practicing physician assistants up to date with current clinical practice by providing timely articles reviewing the state of the art in patient care.

TARGET AUDIENCE

Physician Assistants and other healthcare professionals

LEARNING OBJECTIVES

Upon completion of this activity, participants will be able to:
1. Review the history and evolution of mental health.
2. Discuss behavioral therapy, non-pharmacological, and pharmacological interventions in behavioral and mental health.
3. Recognize specific issues and statistics related to the LGBTQ+ community.

ACCREDITATION

The Elsevier Office of Continuing Medical Education (EOCME) is accredited by the Accreditation Council for Continuing Medical Education (ACCME) to provide continuing medical education for physicians.

The EOCME designates this journal-based CME activity for a maximum of 16 *AMA PRA Category 1 Credit(s)*™. Physicians should claim only the credit commensurate with the extent of their participation in the activity.

All other healthcare professionals requesting continuing education credit for this enduring material will be issued a certificate of participation.

DISCLOSURE OF CONFLICTS OF INTEREST

The EOCME assesses conflict of interest with its instructors, faculty, planners, and other individuals who are in a position to control the content of CME activities. All relevant conflicts of interest that are identified are thoroughly vetted by EOCME for fair balance, scientific objectivity, and patient care recommendations. EOCME is committed to providing its learners with CME activities that promote improvements or quality in healthcare and not a specific proprietary business or a commercial interest.

The planning committee, staff, authors and editors listed below have identified no financial relationships or relationships to products or devices they or their spouse/life partner have with commercial interest related to the content of this CME activity:

Yennie Armand, MS, PA-C; Lee I. Ascherman, MD, MPH; Esther Bennitta; Kary Allyn Blair, BS, MBA; Regina Chavous-Gibson, MSN, RN; Brenda S. Fisher, PA-C, JD; Johanna Greenberg, PA-C, MPAS; Katerina Heidhausen; Rodney Ho, PhD, MPH, PA-C, Psychiatry-CAQ; Shinu Kuriakose, DHSc, PA-C, DFAAPA; Kerrigan LeBoeuf, BSN, RN; Nicole E. Miller, PA-C; Charlene M. Morris, MPAS, PA-C, DFAAPA; Megan E. Pater, MPAS, MA, PA-C; Phyllis R. Peterson, PA-C, MPAS, CAQpsy; Axell Ivan Jade Purificacion; Melissa Rodzen, PA-C; Samantha Salyer, PharmD, MS Ed; Jay C. Somers, MS, PA-C, DFAAPA; Lisa Tannenbaum, PA-C; James A. Van Rhee, MS, PA-C; Kim Zuber, PAC, MS.

The planning committee, staff, authors and editors listed below have identified financial relationships or relationships to products or devices they or their spouse/life partner have with commercial interest related to the content of this CME activity:

Michael Asbach, MPAS, PA-C: Speakers bureau and/or consultant/advisor for AbbVie Inc, Avanir Pharmaceuticals, Inc, Neurocrine Biosciences, Inc, Otsuka America Pharmaceutical, Inc, Jane S. Davis, CRNP, DNP: speakers bureau for Amgen Inc, Robert Sobule, MS, PA-C, CAQ-Psychiatry: consultant/advisor for Alkermes

UNAPPROVED/OFF-LABEL USE DISCLOSURE

The EOCME requires CME faculty to disclose to the participants:
1. When products or procedures being discussed are off-label, unlabelled, experimental, and/or investigational (not US Food and Drug Administration [FDA] approved); and
2. Any limitations on the information presented, such as data that are preliminary or that represent ongoing research, interim analyses, and/or unsupported opinions. Faculty may discuss information about pharmaceutical agents that is outside of FDA-approved labelling. This information is intended solely for CME and is not intended to promote off-label use of these medications. If you have any questions, contact the medical affairs department of the manufacturer for the most recent prescribing information.

TO ENROLL
The CME program is available to all *Physician Assistant Clinics* subscribers at no additional fee. To subscribe to the *Physician Assistant Clinics*, call customer service at 1-800-654-2452 or sign up online at www.physicianassistant.theclinics.com.

METHOD OF PARTICIPATION
In order to claim credit, participants must complete the following:
1. Complete enrolment as indicated above
2. Read the activity
3. Complete the CME Test and Evaluation. Participants must achieve a score of 70% on the test. All CME Tests and Evaluations must be completed online

CME INQUIRIES/SPECIAL NEEDS
For all CME inquiries or special needs, please contact elsevierCME@elsevier.com.

Contributors

CONSULTING EDITOR

JAMES A. VAN RHEE, MS, PA-C
Associate Professor, Program Director, Yale School of Medicine, Yale Physician Assistant Online Program, New Haven, Connecticut

EDITORS

KIM ZUBER, PAC, MS
Executive Director, American Academy of Nephrology PAs, St Petersburg, Florida

JANE S. DAVIS, CRNP, DNP
Division of Nephrology, The University of Alabama at Birmingham, Birmingham, Alabama

AUTHORS

YENNIE ARMAND, MS, PA-C
Assistant Professor, School of Health Professions, New York Institute of Technology, Old Westbury, New York

MICHAEL ASBACH, MPAS, PA-C
Associate Director of Interventional Psychiatry, DENT Neurologic Institute, Amherst, New York

LEE I. ASCHERMAN, MD, MPH
Clinical Professor, Training and Supervising Analyst, Child Supervising Analyst, The University of Alabama at Birmingham, The Cincinnati Psychoanalytic Institute, Birmingham, Alabama

KARY ALLYN BLAIR, BS, MBA
Senior Clinical Department Administrator, Department of Psychiatry, Texas Tech University Health Sciences Center School of Medicine, Adjunct Instructor, Department of Healthcare Administration and Leadership, Texas Tech University Health Sciences Center School of Health Professions, Lubbock, Texas

JANE S. DAVIS, CRNP, DNP
Division of Nephrology, The University of Alabama at Birmingham, Birmingham, Alabama

BRENDA S. FISHER, PA-C, JD
Medical Staff Advent Health Gordon, Associate Member, Virginia Bar Association, Calhoun, Georgia

JOHANNA GREENBERG, PA-C, MPAS
Assistant Professor (Clinical), Department of Family and Preventive Medicine, University of Utah School of Medicine, Salt Lake City, Utah

RODNEY HO, PhD, MPH, PA-C, Psychiatry-CAQ
Adjunct Instructor, University of West Florida, JBSA-Lackland

SHINU KURIAKOSE, DHSc, PA-C, DFAAPA
Associate Professor, School of Health Professions, New York Institute of Technology, Old Westbury, New York

KERRIGAN LEBOEUF, BSN, RN
Executive Director, Floyd Home Care, Member of LHC Group, Calhoun, Georgia

NICOLE E. MILLER, PA-C
Department of Neuropsychiatry, DENT Neurologic Institute, Amherst, New York

CHARLENE M. MORRIS, MPAS, PA-C, DFAAPA
Louisville, Kentucky

MEGAN E. PATER, MPAS, MA, PA-C
Principal Faculty and Assessment Coordinator, Department of Physician Assistant Studies, Mount St Joseph University, Cincinnati, Ohio

PHYLLIS R. PETERSON, PA-C, MPAS, CAQpsy
Associate Faculty/Director, NP/PA Post Graduate Psychiatry Program, Texas Tech University Health Sciences Center, Lubbock, Texas, Retired; Owner/Provider, Psychiatric PA Services, Leander, Texas; Connell & Associates, Killeen, Texas

MELISSA RODZEN, PA-C
NYU Langone Emergency Department, Brooklyn, New York

SAMANTHA SALYER, PharmD, MS Ed
Adjunct Faculty, Emory & Henry College, School of Health Sciences, Marion, Virginia; Staff Pharmacist, Walgreens Company

ROBERT SOBULE, MS, PA-C, CAQ-Psychiatry
Director of PA Psychiatry Fellowship, Department of Psychiatry, University of Missouri School of Medicine, Columbia, Missouri

JAY C. SOMERS, MS, PA-C, DFAAPA
Las Vegas, Nevada

LISA TANNENBAUM, PA-C
Physician Assistant, Victory Recovery Partners (VRP), Massapequa, New York; Bel Air Center for Addictions, Bel Air, Maryland

KIM ZUBER, PAC, MS
Executive Director, American Academy of Nephrology PAs, St Petersburg, Florida

Contents

> The history of mental illness is a saga of misconceptions, cruelty, and mistreatment. Early humans recognized mental illness but did not understand it. Today, we do not fare much better, although treatment of the mentally ill is somewhat improved. This article presents the historical basis of evaluation, diagnosis, and treatment of those considered mentally "insane."

> Cognitive behavior therapy (CBT) is based on the principles that patients' perceptions of stimuli and subsequent response to these stressors can alter their mood. The psychological response varies based on individuals' own coping strategies. CBT often relies on the cooperation of both the provider and the patient in working through stressors, the emotions they invoke, and the optimal route to acknowledge feelings and overcome them. CBT is used in a wide range of psychiatric therapeutic treatments and can also be effective in some severe mental disorders. The goal of CBT is for patients to lead satisfactory lives.

> As prescribing rates for antipsychotics and antidepressants continue to increase, the likelihood of drug interactions also increases. It is important to understand possible drug interactions that can occur for the various drug classes used to treat psychiatric conditions. Many patients also have comorbid conditions making treatment more challenging. It is imperative that providers be able to treat an aging population properly.

> Depression is a chronic illness affecting 18 million people per year. Typically, medications are used as first line to treat and manage depressive symptoms. However, there are many nonpharmacologic interventions, procedures, and lifestyle changes that can be used to augment the effects of medications. Physical activity, dietary changes, psychotherapy, electroconvulsive therapy, and transcranial magnetic stimulation are all examples of nonpharmacologic techniques that have been proved to be beneficial adjuncts to medication therapy to ameliorate symptoms of depression.

and behavioral health and well-being are inextricably connected to happiness, purpose, and physical health with aging. This article reviews the impact of age on several mental and behavioral health factors. Evaluating patients over age 65 for increasing mental and behavioral health deficits involves numerous complex etiologies and comorbidities. There are low-cost and no-cost mitigation strategies that can be implemented to prolong high quality of life in the advancing years.

Personality is a construct all people possess that ultimately directs their actions, inactions, and emotions throughout their lives. An astounding variety of personality traits find different modes of expression across cultures, communities, families, and individuals, but some are expressed to such extremes they become detrimental to function. However, personality disorders are often misunderstood because of an evolving understanding of psychiatric illness and the subjective assessments and historical vocabulary used by to describe personality characteristics and disease. This article reviews personality disorders and their diagnostic criteria, and discusses common misconceptions, stigmas, and treatment options affecting patients with personality disorders.

Anxiety disorders represent the most common psychiatric illnesses worldwide. According to "Mental Health" (Our World in Data), 3.8% of the population is affected at any 1 time, and the US lifetime incident rate is close to 33%, leading to significant direct and indirect medical costs. The dysfunctional response to worry can manifest itself in a wide range, from somatic to behavioral symptoms. Assessment and diagnosis require a thorough work-up and understanding of anxiety disorders. Treatments include pharmacologic and nonpharmacologic interventions.

Psychosis is a condition where one's mind loses touch with reality. It includes a variety of symptoms including, but not limited to, hallucinations and delusions. Although psychosis is a staple in the diagnosis of schizophrenia, psychotic symptoms also can occur in a variety of mental illnesses and other nonpsychiatric conditions. There is robust research into the theories of developing psychotic symptoms in a variety of illnesses. This article provides a better understanding on the etiology of various "classic" symptoms of psychosis, such as a hallucinations and delusions in addition to bringing more awareness of suicide risk associated with psychosis.

Identifying key risk factors in the patient encounter can help further differentiate between a diagnosis of major depressive disorder and bipolar disorder. Both of these disorders have the potential to affect cognitive function, employment status, and interpersonal relationships that significantly impact quality of life. Treating these disorders can be challenging, especially if the patient is misdiagnosed, as certain medications can be ineffective or make symptoms worse. Antidepressants, although having low rates of remission, are still recommended in unipolar depression. Quetiapine, diet, and psychotherapy have been shown consistently to be effective in treating bipolar depression.

With the fifth edition of the Diagnostic and Statistical Manual of Mental Disorders, somatic disorders were moved to a separate chapter. This review of somatic and related disorders begins with a historical perspective of somatization and anxiety, then progresses through categorization within the fifth edition of the Diagnostic and Statistical Manual of Mental Disorders. Each specific disorder is separately reviewed and highlighted for evaluation and treatment.

Altered mental status (AMS) is a common occurrence in hospital settings and carries a wide differential. Identifying causes and treatment plans can be challenging, even for experienced providers. In addition to maintaining detailed knowledge of disease presentations and obtaining a thorough history and physical examination, choosing appropriate vocabulary to reflect the patient's presentation is imperative to guiding management. Although many conditions causing AMS changes may be improved or even resolved in the acute setting, changes in mental status can carry long-term consequences and should be prevented whenever possible.

Mental health care has evolved throughout the years in response to cultural norms, understanding of the disease, and the availability of treatments. The twenty-first century is providing new challenges and opportunities in mental health care. The rapid transition to automation and artificial intelligence is causing economic disruption and is expected to displace up to 30% of the current workforce. As society has become more individualized, people are becoming lonelier, which can lead to adverse health outcomes. Mobile applications and telemedicine provide opportunities to change the way care is delivered to patients, reducing stigma and other barriers to treatment.

PHYSICIAN ASSISTANT CLINICS

FORTHCOMING ISSUES

October 2021
Gastroenterology
Jennifer Eames, *Editor*

January 2022
Preventive Medicine
Stephanie Neary, *Editor*

April 2022
The Kidney
Kim Zuber and Jane S. Davis, *Editors*

RECENT ISSUES

April 2021
Surgery
Courtney Fankhanel, *Editor*

January 2021
Rheumatology
Benjamin J Smith, *Editor*

October 2020
Pediatric Orthopedics
Patrick Parenzin, *Editor*

SERIES OF RELATED INTEREST

Psychiatric Clinics
https://www.psych.theclinics.com/

THE CLINICS ARE AVAILABLE ONLINE!
Access your subscription at:
www.theclinics.com

Preface

Behavioral Health: The Need, the Solution, and the Gap Between

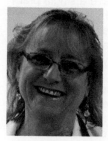 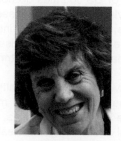

Kim Zuber, PAC, MS   Jane S. Davis, CRNP, DNP
Editors

> *I hate being in groups with the bipolars. You can never get a word in edgewise.*
> *—VA patient with schizophrenia discussing mental health groups*

Mental health permeates all aspects of medicine, from the primary care office to the orthopedic office to the emergency department (ED). Close to 20% of all Americans experienced mental illness in 2018, the last year with complete data.[1] One in 25 Americans experiences serious mental illness. One in 8 ED visits was for mental illness or substance abuse disorders. Looking at the homeless population in the United States, one in 5 homeless Americans has serious mental illness. More than one-third of all incarcerated adults in the United States have a diagnosed mental illness. Mood disorders are the most likely cause of hospitalization in the under-45 age group (excluding pregnancy). Three-quarters of all youth in the juvenile justice system have a diagnosed mental illness. More than 40% of all Veterans Administration (VA) patients have a diagnosed mental illness or substance abuse disorder. Depression is the leading cause of disability worldwide.[1]

These mental health issues affect all aspects of medicine, for example, patients with depression have a 40% higher risk of developing cardiovascular disease.[1] For the US economy, the cost of mental illness is $193.2 billion in lost earnings each year; this does not include the expense of health care, medications, or lost wages from unpaid caregivers. The rate of unemployment for the person with mental illness is 2 times as high as for those without mental illness. High school students with depression are 2 times as likely to drop out of school. Adults with mental illness often experience substance abuse, a 20% incidence in 2019. This leads to a need for caregiving within the family/friends with the expectation of caregivers spending an average of 32 hours a week providing unpaid care.[1] The *"graying"* of America means that the incidence of

Physician Assist Clin 6 (2021) xiii–xv
https://doi.org/10.1016/j.cpha.2021.03.005
2405-7991/21/© 2021 Elsevier Inc. All rights reserved.

physicianassistant.theclinics.com

age-related dementia will continue to increase, and the need for unpaid caregivers will continue to grow.[2] The Centers for Disease Control and Prevention reported that for just 1 week in June 2020, 40% of all Americans stated that they were struggling with mental health or substance abuse issues due to the COVID crisis.[3] The incidence was significantly higher for younger adults, racial/ethnic minorities, essential workers, and unpaid adult caregivers.

While those in need of mental health services is increasing, the number of mental health experts is shrinking. Sixty percent of US counties do not have a single practicing psychiatrist. As many of us know, trying to get a patient seen by a mental health professional can be a game of long waits for appointments, insurance coverage issues, and lack of coverage, and then, due to the underlying issues with the patient, often a missed appointment when you have pulled every string you know how to pull to acquire that appointment.

Physician assistants (PAs) have been involved in mental health issues, originally by default from their origins as medics in the Vietnam War, but more recently as they move to fill the gaps in medical care in the United States.[4] PAs, as medical providers with the ability to care for both the mental and the physical health of patients, would seem to be a logical choice. While the move to mental health/behavioral health care was accepted by the medical community, the insurance industry was less accepting. They wanted proof of expertise and additional training in order to certify PAs as mental health caregivers. The National Commission for Certification of PAs stepped in with a certificate of added qualifications specifically for psychiatry.[5] The VA and military, with their desperate need for mental health experts, also saw PAs as a much-needed bridge to increase mental health providers in the twenty-first century. The Air Force is taking the lead by opening the first postgraduate psychiatric fellowship for active-duty PAs in San Antonio, Texas (Rodney Ho, 2020, personal communication).

Against this backdrop of increasing need, behavioral health experts across the United States have come together to develop a "primer" of what PAs in mental and behavioral health do on a day-to-day basis. We start with an overview of the history of the entire psychiatric profession by Davis and Zuber. Then, we move on to the underpinnings of the need to consider behavioral therapy and other nonpharmacologic interventions and the successes they have had in an article by Kuriakose and Armand. As psychiatric medicine moves more and more to the chemical, Salyer reviews common medications used, telling us where, when, and how, and highlighting both side effects and drug-drug interactions. Miller teaches us how we can treat patients with depression via cognitive behavioral therapy, while Fisher and LeBoeuf highlight legal issues (federal and state specific) we confront while caring for our patients.

Greenberg discusses the specific issues and statistics in the lesbian, gay, bisexual, transgender, and queer+ (LGBTQ+) community. Since youths in the LGBTQ+ community are more than 4 times more likely to attempt suicide, and often succeed, this is a group that warrants the attention of all PAs. Blair shows us the issues with outpatient care for psychiatric care, including how we have come to a time in our history where the vast majority of homeless have mental health issues. Ascherman teaches us the special and important issues regarding children and mental health, highlighting the suicide rate of American's youth. Somers and Morris discuss mental health and the elderly, a growing issue and vitally important to those in practice. Tannenbaum and Rodzen tell us about personality disorders, while Peterson and Ho discuss anxiety. Ho also does a detailed piece about posttraumatic stress disorder (PTSD) and the newest diagnosis and treatment of this common finding. Sobule highlights psychotic disorders and all their differences. Pater breaks down unipolar, bipolar, and all the permutations of these disorders. Peterson tells us about somatic disorders; those of you in primacy care and emergency medicine are the most likely to see this presentation in your practice. Rodzen and Tannenbaum discuss the presentation of dementia versus delirium, a HUGE issue in the hospitalized patient that often complicates the medical care of inpatients. We finish with Asbach discussing loneliness and isolation. While this issue of *Physician Assistant Clinics* was developed long before COVID hit the front pages of everything we see and do, Asbach's topic has taken on a new immediacy in 2021.

We hope you enjoy this issue as much as we enjoyed pulling it together. We thank all our authors, but we especially thank Scott Richards, PAC and Director of the Monmouth, New Jersey PA program. Without his wisdom and expertise, we would never have been able to put this special issue of *Physician Assistant Clinics* "Behavioral Medicine" together.

Kim Zuber, PAC, MS
American Academy of Nephrology PAs
131 31st Avenue
St Petersburg, FL 33704, USA

Jane S. Davis, CRNP, DNP
Division of Nephrology
University of Alabama at Birmingham
Birmingham, AL 35294, USA

E-mail addresses:
zuberkim@yahoo.com (K. Zuber)
jsdavis@uabmc.edu (J.S. Davis)

REFERENCES

1. National Alliance on Mental Illness. Mental health by the numbers. Arlington, VA. Available at: https://nami.org/mhstats. Accessed August 1, 2020.
2. Centers for Disease Control and Prevention. The state of mental health and aging in America. 2018. Available at: https://www.cdc.gov/aging/pdf/mental_health.pdf?fbclid=IwAR2K-CtioOreiGYNe-FZbCkLWQ54BYfOF61a6ON36-xYue2SASt71qlzSeU. Accessed August 16, 2020.
3. Czeisler MÉ, Lane RI, Petrosky E, et al. Mental health, substance use, and suicidal ideation during the COVID-19 pandemic—United States, June 24–30, 2020. MMWR Morb Mortal Wkly Rep 2020;69:1049–57.
4. Trumbo J. PAs perfect bridge between medical and mental health. AAPA Web site. Available at: https://www.aapa.org/news-central/2017/04/pas-perfect-bridge-vetween-medical-mental-health/. Accessed August 9, 2020.
5. Specialty certificates of added qualifications (CAQ). NCCPA Web site. Available at: https://www.nccpa.net/Specialty-CAQs. Accessed August 9, 2020.

The Historical Landscape of Mental Health Evaluation and Treatment

Jane S. Davis, CRNP, DNP[a,1], Kim Zuber, PAC, MS[b],*

KEYWORDS

- Mental health • Hysteria • Trepanning • DSM • Housing the insane
- Mental health treatments

KEY POINTS

- The history of mental health is a saga of misunderstanding and lack of insight with progress lagging behind other specialties.
- Treatments have ranged from brutality to medications.
- Our mental health system is understaffed, overburdened, and underfunded.
- The *Diagnostic and Statistical Manual*, now in its fifth edition, provides a groundwork for diagnosing and treating behavioral issues.

INTRODUCTION

Historically, the story of perceptions, beliefs, and treatment of mental illness is a tale worthy of a Stephen King novel. Sadly, it is not a novel but a true story. The understanding of mental health has evolved from possession by evil spirits to genetics to modern-day medicine. Only by looking back to see where we have been can we realize how different our evaluation and treatment of behavioral issues are in 2021. No longer do we drive holes into skulls to release "bad spirits," sacrifice virgins on altars, or "bleed" patients to remove "bad humors," but instead we attempt to isolate the brain abnormalities and treat the specific type of mental illness. Is this progress? We have patients living on the streets, unable to care for themselves, while we tell ourselves it is their choice. Is this progress?

During a mental health crisis, the patient is more likely to be arrested rather than taken to a psychiatric care center. Each year more than 2 million patients with mental health issues are jailed. Close to 15% of the men and 30% of the women in prisons

Potential Conflicts of Interest: Dr J. Davis is on the Amgen Speakers Bureau. Both authors were responsible for the research, development, and writing of the article.
[a] Division of Nephrology, University of Alabama at Birmingham; [b] American Academy of Nephrology PAs
[1] Present address: 3605 Oakdale Rd, Birmingham, AL 35223.
* Corresponding author. 131 31st Avenue, St Petersburg, FL 33704.
E-mail address: zuberkim@yahoo.com

Physician Assist Clin 6 (2021) 361–369
https://doi.org/10.1016/j.cpha.2021.02.001
2405-7991/21/© 2021 Elsevier Inc. All rights reserved.

physicianassistant.theclinics.com

have a serious mental health issue.[1] These percentages are considered a low estimate, as many of these patients are incorrectly diagnosed.[2] In fact, prisons are often referred to as the largest mental health institute in the United States, if not the world.[3] Patients with mental illness are often incarcerated longer and abused within the jails. Frequently, they are released and left to fend for themselves without any treatment or follow-up. One-third of the homeless are estimated to have a serious mental illness, but studies in specific localities show even higher estimates. For example, a 2007 study in Roanoke, Virginia showed 70% of the homeless have mental illness, whereas a study in 2009 showed 67% of the homeless in Colorado Springs had mental illness.[4,5]

MENTAL HEALTH IN EARLY TIMES

Early humans believed mental illness was the result of evil spirits. The lack of understanding and social stigma are still prevalent today. Skulls dating back as far as 5000 BCE show evidence of holes bored through the bone (trephining or trepanning; **Fig. 1**). Trephining or trepanning was thought to allow evil spirits to escape the body. In actuality, drill holes were helpful for those patients with intracranial bleeds, so the good response in this subgroup helped early practitioners continue using the "treatment."[6]

In the sixth century BCE, Egyptian papyri were found that recommended music and recreational activities, such as dancing, as a relief for mental illness. It is interesting that we use very similar treatments for some of our patients with dementia today.[6]

Later, the Greeks dismissed the supernatural basis for illness and focused instead on the imbalance of the 4 humors: blood, bile, black bile, and phlegm. Treatments ranged from purging to bloodletting to special diets.[6]

Attitudes toward the mentally ill have run the gamut from family care to abandonment. Women have always had a special place in the history of mental health treatment. It is no coincidence that the Greek term *hyster* for uterus and hysteria have

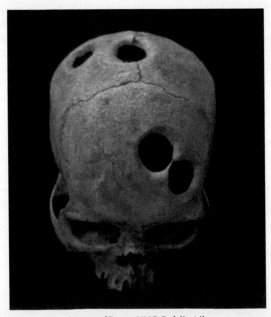

Fig. 1. Trephining in ancient cultures. (*From* NYC Public Library; open access.)

the same root. In the second century when hysteria was first described, it was considered to affect women only. The Egyptians believed the source of hysteria was the movement of the uterus with the repositioning the organ to be the cure. Interesting enough, sexual activity culminating in orgasm was often the treatment. It was not until the late nineteenth century when Freud published his book, *Studies on Hysteria*, that hysteria was viewed as being neurologic in origin and experienced by men as well.[7]

One of the first known mental hospitals opened in 792 CE in Baghdad (**Fig. 2**). Islam taught that the mentally ill were deserving of humane treatment. Avicenna of Arabia, a Persian philosopher, is credited as the founder. His most famous books, *The Canon of Medicine* and *The Book of Healing*, were used by universities and scholars to treat patients and remained in use in use until 1650.[8]

Witches were often blamed for the world's ills from crop failures to plagues to locusts. When disasters occurred, a cause had to identified. Women bore more than their share of persecution. *Joan of Arc* and the *Salem Witch Trials* are the most famous, but they were by no means isolated incidents. Although many of the "witches" of the seventeenth and eighteenth centuries are now presumed to have had mental illness, witch hunts were also used to dispose of those not wanted by society. By the time witch hunts declined, more than 100,000 women had been burned at the stake.[6]

Religion and mental health have been intertwined since the origins of mankind. From beliefs that those with mental issues were being "punished" or were "possessed by demons" to the Hindu concept that the 4 areas of life must be in balance, religious beliefs have often dictated treatment of those with mental illness.[9]

HOUSING OF THE "INSANE"

Workhouses and asylums were opened to house (not necessarily to care for) the mentally ill or those thought to be mentally ill. Oftentimes, the conditions were abusive and inhumane. In addition to bloodletting and purging, patients were often doused with either very hot or cold water (a precursor to water boarding).[10] In 1792, Philippe Pinel focused on kindness and care as treatment. He cleaned the Paris *Hospice de*

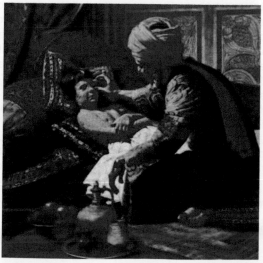

Fig. 2. Baghdad Mental Hospital. (*From* NYC Public Library; open access.)

Bicetre, removed chains, and allowed patients free movement.[6] An English Quaker, William Tuke, using Pinel's methods, established a facility for mental health, *The York Retreat*, that has been in existence for more than 200 years.[10]

Unfortunately, not all institutions were so benign. *Bethlem Royal Hospital*, colloquially referred to as *Bedlam*, was founded in 1247.[11] Because of financial issues, transfers of the hospital back and forth between the state and the religious order occurred. Bedlam reverted into housing for the criminally insane by the early 1900s. Inmates were often chained to the wall and left to lie in their excrement. In order to finance these institutions, fees were charged, as spectators came to view the patients.[12]

In the United States, Benjamin Rush, often referred to as the "founder of American psychiatry" and a co-signer of the Declaration of Independence, was an early proponent of "heroic depletion therapy," which included bloodletting, purging with active mercury, and shock for a "humeral imbalance."[13] Rush developed a "tranquilizing chair," which combined centrifugal force and injections of tranquilizers until the patient threw up, became quiet, or apologized for bad behavior.[14] Although some of his methods were barbaric from our point of view, he also advocated for humane housing for those with mental illness, treatment of addiction, and the concept that mental illness is a disease.[15]

Although women often suffered the most from mistreatment and persecution, 2 women in particular are at the forefront of humane treatment and understanding of mental illness. In nineteenth century America, Dorothea Dix took up the cause for better treatment and understanding of mental illness.[16] The mid 1800s was a time ripe for reform. In addition to the abolitionists, there were multiple other movements. Dix herself experienced what we now know was clinical depression, which was treated by a Grand Tour of Europe (a treatment popular with upper classes). While there, she fell under the influence of popular reformers.[16]

After returning to America, Dix was teaching a Sunday school class in a prison and was appalled at the treatment of the mentally ill, who were often unclothed, underfed, and chained to walls in the cold. "*Lunatics cannot feel the cold*" was the explanation of one of the jailers. Dix took up the cause of reform and, influenced by European ideas, she promoted a healthy environment for the mentally ill. By 1880, she had helped establish 30 of the first 123 institutions in North America.[16]

In the United States, mental institutions were often hidden away, and abuse was common. Nellie Bly, one of the first "girl stunt reporters," shocked the world by her exposé of life in a mental hospital (**Fig. 3**).[17] In 1817, she feigned madness in order to be committed to the Women's Lunatic Asylum on Blackwell's Island, New York. Nellie went in not knowing when or even if she would be released. Her 10 days made front page news for *The New York World* and enough material for a book (*Ten Days in a Madhouse*). The inmates were doused with cold water and made to sit for hours on wooden benches without talking or moving. The food was rancid and inedible. The inmates were abused and tortured (again water boarding was a frequent occurrence).[17]

Nellie Bly paved the way for other girl reporters, and she continued her undercover work as an unwed mother, chorus girl, and servant. She is also known for having circled the world in 72 days, beating the time from Jules Verne's popular story.[17]

MENTAL HEALTH IN THE TWENTIETH CENTURY

By the end of the nineteenth century, there was a movement to attribute mental illness to somatic origins. There were multiple schools of thought of psychotherapy (some estimate more than 400 different approaches), including hypnosis, later followed by psychotherapy.[6]

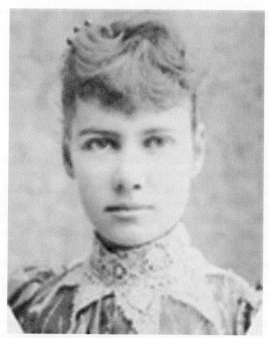

Fig. 3. Nellie Bly. (*From* NYC Public Library; open access.)

The father of psychoanalysis theory, Sigmund Freud, was influential at the turn of the twentieth century.[18,19] His concepts of the id, the ego, the superego, repression of the unconscious, and the subconscious still infuse treatment of mental illness in the twenty-first century.[6]

In the 1930s, lobotomies were seen as the answer for many conditions, including schizophrenia, severe depression, and bipolar disorder.[7] The process of a lobotomy is quick and easy, resulting in docile patients following the procedure. The downside is the radical change to the personality.

In the United States, until the late 1970s, restraints, shock therapy, and lobotomies continued to be standard until the introduction of medication and the view that mental illness was a chemical imbalance. Western psychologists researched cognitive approaches to behavioral health while identifying mental illness as a disease to be approached similarly as any other disease state.[10] Electroconvulsive therapy, commonly referred to as "shock therapy," is still used today. However, it is used under more controlled conditions and anesthesia than was initially practiced. The movie, *One Flew Over the Cuckoo's Nest*, famously depicted both shock therapy and lobotomies and their effects on patients.

THE *DIAGNOSTIC AND STATISTICAL MANUAL*

Although many believe that the classification system developed and used for the *Diagnostic and Statistical Manual* (DSM) was due to a growth in psychiatry, it is not quite true. The original impetus was the US Census.[20,21] In 1840, the census collected statistical information on "idiocy/insanity," but the data were flawed. Some towns listed all African Americans as "idiots," while others listed blindness or deafness as "insanity." Frederick Wines authored a report on the "Defective, Dependent and Delinquent

Classes of the population of the United States" using the data from the 1880 census where he used 7 categories of mental illness20,21:

- Dementia
- Dipsomania (uncontrollable craving for alcohol)
- Epilepsy
- Mania
- Melancholia
- Monomania
- Paresis

These same categories were used by Emil Kraepelin in 1883 when he published a system of psychological disorders organized around symptoms. Again, this was used in 1917 for a collection of standardized data collected by all the mental hospitals in the United States.[21] These data morphed into the first edition of the American Medical Associations Standard Classified Nomenclature of Disease or *"The Standard."*[22] This classification system was developed and used for inpatients with severe psychiatric disorders.

In 1942, during World War II, Army psychiatrists developed a classification system for outpatients that was adopted by the entire US military complex and Veterans Association.[23] This system was referred to as *Medical 203* and formed the basis for the first *DSM*.

DSM-I was published in 1952 at 130 pages and with 106 mental disorders, including *"personality disorders."*[24] Homosexuality was listed as a psychiatric disorder in this initial edition. In the 1960s, the concept of psychiatric illness was undergoing a societal change. The *DSM-II* (1968) was difficult to use in clinical practice. One study showed trained psychiatrists could not agree on a *DSM* diagnosis when presented with the same patient.[25] Influenced by gay rights activists who inserted themselves into the 1970 American Psychiatric Association (APA) conference in San Francisco, research from Kinsey and Hooker on sexuality in the United States, and articles decrying the reliability of the *DSM*, the next printing of the *DSM* listed homosexuality as a *"sexual orientation disturbance."*[26,27]

In 1974, a committee led by Robert Spitzer[25] sought to align the *DSM* with the *International Statistical Classification of Diseases* codes. The result was a huge rescaling of diagnoses. Spitzer and Fleiss[27] used the draft version for 2 years to confirm its usefulness in both diagnosis and treatment. There was an issue with the removal of neuroses, but with the return of that diagnosis code, the APA published *DSM-III* in 1980. This version had 265 diagnostic codes and was 494 pages long with claims made regarding its reliability based on the field tests from the 1970s. The *DSM-III* was considered a revolution in psychiatry and was used both nationally and internationally.

That is not to say that revisions and updates were not needed. *DSM-III* was revised in 1987; *DSM-IV*, published in 1994, was revised in 2000, and *DSM-V* was published in 2013. Although the *DSM* has helped practitioners diagnose and treat mental and behavioral illness, facilitating insurance reimbursement, it is not without its warts. Relying on western culture and with its multitude of disorders, it is estimated that using its criteria, almost half of all Americans could be diagnosed with a psychiatric disorder in their lifetimes.[6]

THE RISE OF MEDICATIONS

Although various drugs and potions had been used for treatment, the use of medications for the treatment of mental health became commonplace in the twentieth century. Lithium is a naturally occurring element with antidotes of lithium used in Denmark in the 1800s with success in psychiatric issues. In 1949, John Cade[28] was the first to publish data showing the effectiveness of lithium in the treatment of acute mania. In the 1940s and 1950s, antihistamines were developed. Their side effects of sleepiness and sedation became the basis of neuroleptics developed and used for treatment of schizophrenia.[29] Chlorpromazine, marketed as *Thorazine* in the United States, was introduced the early 1950s and promoted as the most effective treatment for schizophrenia.[30]

Medications including opium, cocaine, barbiturates, and valium came and went as medications of choice for psychiatric disorders.[31] Amphetamines and narcotics were developed and used with protocols and diagnoses changing treatment concepts throughout the twentieth and twenty-first centuries. Although the vast array of medications has greatly improved treatment and life for countless patients, they have brought with them the dark side of overuse, abuse, and addiction.[32]

In the 1950s and 1960s, the Central Intelligence Agency (CIA) became interested in *"mind control"* and using psychotropic medications. The infamous *Project MK-Ultra* occurred from 1953 to 1973 with the participation (sometimes unwittingly) of 150 human subjects to psychedelic drugs, paralytics, and/or electroshock therapy.[32] This program expanded to experimentation with LSD (lysergic acid diethylamide) at Stanford, University, Columbia, University, and Harvard University. Out of these experiments came many famous 1960s counterculture names: CIA chemist Sidney Gottlieb, *One Flew over the Cuckoo's Nest* author Ken Kesey, Unabomber Ted Kaczynski, and psychology professor Timothy Leary, among others. These experiments also led to the publication of President Ford's Executive Order requiring "informed consent" for all test subjects.[32] In 2019, it was estimated that 1 in 6 Americans took a psychotropic medication.[33] This estimate did not include those who self-treated with either over-the-counter medications and/or legal or illegal drugs, such as marijuana (the legality of which varies from state to state).

In the 1960s, the concept of a monoamine hypothesis (depletion of serotonin, norepinephrine, and dopamine) was developed, and the first medications were introduced.[34] The monoamine hypothesis also led to the development of antidepressant medications and classes, from monoamine oxidase inhibitors to tricyclic antidepressants to selective serotonin reuptake inhibitors to serotonin-norepinephrine reuptake inhibitors to atypical antidepressants to antianxiety medications. Medications for treatment of behavioral issues became standard for a variety of conditions. However, in the twenty-first century, we are seeing a swing back to nonmedication cognitive behavioral treatment and less dependence on pharmacology.

SUMMARY

This history of civilization and mental illness, abuse, and compassion are intertwined. In retrospect, treatments seem like a pendulum widely swinging from one side to the other. Today, we pride ourselves on our understanding and our knowledge of the chemistry involved in the neurologic system. We can tailor treatments to a person's genetic code and choose from a wide range of options, pharmacologic and nonpharmacologic. At the same time, the mentally ill are often incarcerated with little or no treatment. Shabby unkempt men and women roam our streets. The drug hailed as a breakthrough today is abused next week and reviled the week after. We have found solutions to many problems, but as each problem appears to be solved, another takes its place, posing new challenges and forcing us the reexamine our treatments and understanding.

REFERENCES

1. National Alliance on Mental Illness, Arlington, VA. Available at: https://www.nami.org/Advocacy/Policy-Priorities/Divert-from-Justice-Involvement/Jailing-People-with-Mental-Illness. Accessed May 1, 2020.

2. Martin MS, Haynes K, Hatcher S, et al. Diagnostic error in correctional mental health: prevalence, causes, and consequences. J Correct Health Care 2016; 22(2):109–17.

3. Al-Rousan T, Rubenstein L, Sieleni B, et al. Inside the nation's largest mental health institution: a prevalence study in a state prison system. BMC Public Health 2017;17(1):342.

4. Treatment Advocacy Center (TAC). How many individuals with a serious mental illness are homeless – backgrounder. 2016. Available at: http://www.treatmentadvocacycenter.org/problem/consequences-of-non-treat. Accessed May 1, 2020.

5. Available at: https://www.psychologytoday.com/us/blog/beyond-schizophrenia/201608/homeless-mentally-ill-and-neglected. Accessed May 1, 2020.

6. Farreras IG. History of mental illness. General psychology required reading. 2019. Available at: https://www.academia.edu/26494009/History_of_mental_illness. Accessed April 26, 2020.

7. Foerschener AM. The history of mental illness from skull drills to happy pills. Inquiries J 2010;2(9):4. Available at: http://www.inquiriesjournal.com/articles/1673/3/the-history-of-mental-illness-from-skull-drills-to-happy-pills. Accessed April 26, 2020.

8. Saffari M, Pakpour A. Avicenna's Canon of Medicine: a look at health, public health, and environmental sanitation. Arch Iran Med 2012;15(12):785–9.

9. Wig NN. Mental health and spiritual values. A view from the east. Int Rev Psychiatry 1999;11:92–6.

10. Butcher JN, Mineka S, Hooley JM. Abnormal psychology (16th ed.) 2014.

11. Briggs A, Porter R, Tucker P, et al. The history of Bethlem. London: Psychology Press; 1997.

12. Andrews J. Bedlam Revisited: a history of Bethlem hospital c.1634 – c.1770 [PhD thesis]. London: Queen Mary and Westfield College, London University; 1991.

13. Shorter, Edward (1997). A history of psychiatry: from the era of the asylum to the age of Prozac. Wiley.

14. Beam, Alex (2001). Gracefully insane: life and death inside America's premier mental hospital.

15. North RL. Benjamin Rush, MD: assassin or beloved healer?". Proc Bayl Univ Med Cent 2000;13(1):45–9.

16. Strickler J, Farmer T. Dorothy Dix: crusader for patients with mental illness. Nursing 2019;49(1):49–510.

17. Bernard D. She went undercover to expose an insane asylum's horrors. Now Nellie Bly is getting her due. Washington Post. 7/28/19. Available at: https://www.washingtonpost.com/history/2019/07/28/she-went-undercover-expose-an-insane-asylums-horrors-now-nellie-bly-is-getting-her-due/. Accessed May 28, 2020.

18. Jones E. What is psychoanalysis? London: Allen & Unwin; 1949. p. 47.

19. Mannoni O. Freud: the theory of the unconscious. London: Verso; 2015.

20. South SC, DeYoung NJ. Behavior genetics of personality disorders: informing classification and conceptualization in DSM-5. Personal Disord 2013;4(3):270–83.

21. American Psychiatric Association (APA), History of the DSM. Available at: https://www.psychiatry.org/psychiatrists/practice/dsm/history-of-the-dsm. Accessed May 9, 2020.
22. Greenberg SA, Shuman DW, Meyer RG. Unmasking forensic diagnosis. Int J L Psychiatry 2004;27(1):1–15.
23. Houts AC. Fifty years of psychiatric nomenclature: reflections on the 1943 War Department Technical Bulletin, Medical 203. J Clin Psychol 2000;56(7):935–67.
24. Grob GN. Origins of DSM-I: a study in appearance and reality. Am J Psychiatry 1991;148(4):421–31.
25. Spitzer RL, Fleiss JL. A re-analysis of the reliability of psychiatric diagnosis. Br J Psychiatry 1974;125(0):341–7.
26. Dresher J. Out of DSM: Depathologizing Homosexuality. Behav Sci 2015;5: 565–75.
27. Spitzer RL. The diagnostic status of homosexuality in DSM-III: a reformulation of the issues. Am J Psychiatry 1981;138(2):210–5.
28. Cade JF. John Frederick Joseph Cade: family memories on the occasion of the 50th anniversary of his discovery of the use of lithium in mania, 1949. Aust N Z J Psychiatry 1999;33(5):615–22.
29. Chopko TC, Lindsley CW. Classics in chemical neuroscience: risperidone. ACS Chem Neurosci 2018;9(7):1520–9.
30. Capenter WT, Koenig JI. The evolution of drug development in schizophrenia: past issues and future opportunities. Neuropsychopharmacology 2008;33(9): 2061–79.
31. Coomber R, McElrath K, Measham F, et al. Key concepts in drugs and society (SAGE Key concepts series). 1st edition. London: SAGE Publications Ltd; 2013.
32. History.com Editors. MK-Ultra. History. 2018. Available at: https://www.history.com/topics/us-government/history-of-mk-ultra. Accessed May 17, 2020.
33. Braslow JT, Marder SR. History of psychopharmacology. Annu Rev Clin Psychol 2019;15:25–50.
34. Hillhouse TM, Porter JH. A brief history of the development of antidepressant drugs: from monoamines to glutamate. Exp Clin Psychopharmacol 2015; 23(1):1–21.

Cognitive Behavior Therapy
Patient-Centered, Timely, and Effective Paradigm

Shinu Kuriakose, DHSc, PA-C, DFAAPA*, Yennie Armand, MS, PA-C

KEYWORDS

- Cognitive behavior therapy • Quality of life • Dysfunctional thoughts
- Patient commitment • Short-term • Gold standard • Mood validation

KEY POINTS

- Cognitive Behavioral Therapy is viewed as the gold standard in for specific cases of depression and anxiety.
- CBT is often used in an adjunct manner with antidepressant medications as appropriate.
- Optimally, CBT involves a partnership between providers and their patients.

HISTORY AND DEVELOPMENT OF COGNITIVE BEHAVIOR THERAPY

Throughout recorded history, many civilizations have identified the scientific study of psychology as fundamental to the functioning and behavior of individuals. As scientific experts throughout history have studied mental disorder (the abnormality of psychological functioning), they have classified it into distinct domains of biological, psychodynamic, behavioral, cognitive, and humanistic factors. Behavioral therapy's first influencers were Ivan Pavlov, John B. Watson, B.F. Skinner, John Dollard, Neal Miller, and Joseph Wolpe in the early 1900s, who concluded that classical and operant conditioning could change human behavior.[1] Rational emotive behavior therapy was established as a psychological approach for the treatment of psychosocial disorders in the 1950s thanks to its founder, Dr Albert Ellis.[2] The cognitive behavioral field was received with great criticism in its infancy stage in the 1960s because of the empirical belief that cognition was not an observable form and could not produce measurable data. Dr Aaron Beck, who is regarded as the father of cognitive therapy (CT), initially rejected the concept of CT himself until the late 1970s, when his research concluded

Funding: None.
Conflicts of interest: No conflict of interest.
School of Health Professions, New York Institute of Technology, Northern Boulevard, Old Westbury, NY 11568, USA
* Corresponding author.
E-mail address: Skuria06@nyit.edu

that the development of depression is cognitive. Beck's Model of Depression, also termed the cognitive triad, described the theory that thoughts influence behavior and that maladaptive thinking styles lead to maladaptive behaviors and emotional distress. In other words, cognition influences emotions and influences behavior.[3] The psychological models that merged to create the concept of cognitive behavior therapy (CBT) are those that were traditionally separate entities: behavioral therapy and CT. It was not imagined that these contradictory therapies would ever prove to be complimentary. CBT initially showed positive clinical outcomes in the treatment of phobias, which quickly expanded its use in the treatment of personality disorders in the 1980s. CBT is now one of the most used forms of psychotherapy.[3]

SIGNIFICANCE TO PATIENTS WITH MENTAL ILLNESS

As with depression, a vast array of treatment modalities, including pharmacotherapy, electroconvulsive therapy (ECT), and psychotherapy, have been theorized and challenged for the management and treatment of most mental illnesses. Depending on the severity and nature of a disorder, a single treatment modality poses limitations to its success. Integrating the fundamentals of behavioral and cognitive models, clinicians can better understand how emotions, beliefs, and behavior all interrelate in CBT. This understanding has facilitated its application in a wider range of mental disorders that were once limited to pharmacotherapy, cognitive, or behavioral techniques alone.[4] In addition to depression, CBT has offered options for those with panic disorder with or without agoraphobia, generalized anxiety disorder, social phobia, irritable bowel syndrome (IBS), chronic pain, and eating disorders, among many others. It has been considered first-line therapy for posttraumatic stress disorder (PTSD) from supportive research concluding short-term and long-term efficacy exists. When used in conjunction with pharmacotherapy, CBT has lessened the positive and negative symptoms in the management of schizophrenia.

The goal of these principles is to allow clinicians and patients to have a roadmap of how to proceed in a time-conscious, effective, and patient-centric manner. Clinicians have to ensure that patients feel comfortable during this journey of self-revelation and vulnerability on the part of the patients, whereas the patients need to maximize the time spent during a treatment session with the CBT coach and be vested in their "homework" and the true nature of their feelings (**Box 1**). It remains imperative that this roadmap based on these principles be transparent to the patients on initiation of therapy and the patient is given opportunities to explore each of these guideposts robustly. Clinicians need to quantify the time spent in therapy but also ensure that the quality of therapy does lead to measurable positive outcomes. Therefore, a successful CBT paradigm of treatment relies on open communication between the therapist and patient, transparency, time consciousness, and vested interests of both parties in the outcome goals of treatment.[5]

Cognitive Behavior Therapy Remains Fluid and Is Molded by the Patient's Perception of Problems Encountered, Which Are Translated into Cognitive Terms

A core principle of CBT is the dysfunctional and negative thinking by the patient when faced with stressors. Different people can face similar stressors but have varying reactions to them. Coping strategies in the perception of these stressors and mechanisms to overcome the barrier in front of them can help mitigate feelings of being overwhelmed and helpless. CBT clinicians must start by initially scrutinizing the patient's specific thinking process that leads to the current mental health condition. The second step is to explore whether these dysfunctional feelings lead to behaviors

---

Box 1
Fundamental principles of cognitive behavior therapy

As with many therapeutic paradigms, CBT is based on 10 fundamental principles:

CBT is based on an ever-evolving formulation of the patients and their problems in cognitive terms.

CBT requires a good client-therapist relationship

CBT emphasizes collaboration and active participation

CBT is goal oriented and problem focused

CBT initially emphasizes the present

CBT is educative; it aims to teach the clients to be their own therapists and emphasizes relapse prevention

CBT aims to be time limited

CBT sessions are structured

CBT teaches patients to identify, evaluate, and respond to their dysfunctional thoughts and beliefs

CBT uses a variety of techniques to change thinking, mood, and behavior

Adapted from Cognitive Therapy: Basics and Beyond (J. Becks).[5]

---

that are not helpful to the patient. In conversation with the patients, the clinician tries to expose any underlying stressors or experiences undergone in the past that might lead to this current dysfunctional feeling. The past is not a focus of CBT but only a way to recognize that the patient's past journey can color future experiences.[6] The clinician must focus on the patient's perception of stressors in a historical context and the patient's attitude and drive when dealing with these challenges. There might be opportunities for the patient to overcome the negative ways of thinking if the therapist can reframe the patient's perceptions in a cognitive conceptual model. The patient learns to recognize how faulty thinking may lead to negative outcomes, feelings, and subsequent actions; this is a vicious circle that needs to be avoided.

An Authentic Relationship Between the Patient and Therapist Is the Bedrock of Cognitive Behavior Therapy

Transparency, open communication, and mutual trust remain the fundamental bedrock of a good patient-therapist alliance, and it is often the ingredient that leads to positive mental health outcomes. The responsibility of the therapist involves developing a rapport with the patient, validating feelings stemming from stressful situations, and using active listening techniques. The therapist does not necessarily need to agree with the patient's perception but should make an effort to recognize the changes these stressors can have on the patient's mental state; relationships with their friends and family; and the effects on their social, work, and home life. CBT is an evolving treatment strategy where the techniques used might vary based on the presenting symptoms of the patient, but fundamental is a warm, safe, nonjudgmental, and welcoming environment. Talk-back is helpful if the patient hears from the therapist the concerns the patient is voicing, because this increases the patient's comfort by realizing that the therapist is hearing the patient and understands the patient's concerns. It is also prudent to point out small therapeutic successes achieved by the patient when using CBT techniques taught by the therapist. This approach enhances the patient's use of these methods in a more consistent manner. In addition, feedback from the patient on an ongoing basis at the end of the session can help the therapist pivot care in the manner most productive for the patient.

Transparency, Collaboration, and Active Participation Remain Paramount

CBT is time limited, and both the therapist and the patient remain active participants during their journey. Initially, when patients come for treatment, they need more therapeutic care and modalities for altering their dysfunctional thinking and subsequent responses. In the early days of therapy, therapists played an active guide role in teaching patients techniques and helping them focus on their stressors and responses.[7] As therapy progresses, this process must become more collaborative, with the goal that the patients are now able to take more control of their care and help lead the therapist to areas where the patient feels less able to deal with stressors. There might be homework assigned by the therapist, which involves the patients writing down the different stressors faced during their day, old ones or newly encountered, and their response to them. The patients are encouraged to elaborate on these feelings in a written form in a diary and to discuss these thoughts and responses during subsequent visits for treatment. This technique allows the therapist an opportunity to focus and customize care more specifically on the patient's needs while allowing the patient to leave the session with a practical and structured plan in hand. These homework assignments might vary every week based on the improvements seen and shown on the patient's part and therefore the treatment can move on to other residual challenges. As therapy progresses, CBT does involve collaboration, communication, and active participation between the patient and therapist because this relationship has a mutual goal: the patient's well-being.

Focused Achievement of the Goal Is Key

CBT has differed from the traditional concepts and practices of psychoanalytic psychotherapy, also known as Freudian therapy. There is less emphasis on childhood feelings, reflections on upbringing during the early years, and parental response to patients' needs as an infant or child. Freudian therapy, by its very nature, can take several years to reach its conclusion, and some subsets of this treatment are lifelong. CBT focusses more on the behavioral aspects of psychotherapy and developing emotional responses and practical steps to specific stressors. CBT is focused on effective management of symptoms or behaviors, using a time-limited basis, usually 8 to 15 sessions, depending on the situation. Certainly, the patient may develop further symptoms, such as regression of cognitive skills to overcome emotional barriers or unexpected emotional challenges, which may lead to further treatment protocols. During the initial meeting of a CBT session, the therapist and patient must reach a mutual understanding of the cognitive issues that need to be challenged and priority given to techniques to overcome these obstacles. The patient must focus on these techniques daily and report back to the clinician during the next session on progress using these modalities. The therapist might assign practical exercises for the patient that might help the patient realize that the negative cognitive thought process the patient was experiencing did not occur as expected. Frequent positive experiences after engaging in these exercises might help the patient overcome the distorted thinking and lead to long-term productive outcomes.

Cognitive Behavior Therapy Does not Involve Regression into the Past but Focusses on the Present

The emphasis on specific current problems and unhelpful emotional response to stimuli and the subsequent pragmatic therapeutic techniques to overcome these barriers remains crucial in CBT psychosocial techniques. It is valuable to have the patient reiterate these techniques on an ongoing basis during sessions because regression may occur if barriers seem unsurmountable to the patient, especially if these challenges have been present for a long time. Positive outcomes to therapeutic techniques will be seen on a steady basis, which provides positive reinforcement to the patient on overcoming challenges. There are times when dwelling on or emphasizing some aspects of the patient's childhood may play a part in their current treatment regimen. The patient may bring up prior life experiences which the patient believes affects their current situation. At other times, the therapist might decide there is a benefit to having the patient look back to understand where some of these dysfunctional thoughts originate. An example is a patient who was emotionally, physically, and/or sexually abused as a child and the subsequent lack of trust hinders the formation of meaningful relationships as an adult. This situation may have brought the patient to therapy initially, and therefore looking back at the past may play an important role in validating current feelings. There are certain psychiatric diagnoses, such as PTSD, substance abuse, eating disorders, and personality disorders, for which patients seek care. In these cases, it may behoove the clinician and patient to recognize previous trauma and adopt cognitive techniques to tackle present issues rooted in the past.

Cognitive Behavior Therapy Empowers Patients to Take an Active Role in the Care and Focus on Relapse Prevention

Beginning with the first session, the patient and therapist meet, discuss specific issues leading to therapy, find common ground on how to proceed, and discuss the therapeutic process. The work of the patient and therapist during CBT focuses on the significance of people's thoughts and how they affect their actions, and the vicious cycle that this can create. The patient must feel comfortable to openly discuss thoughts with the clinician and the clinician must ensure that the patient does feel safe and welcome. The clinician ensures that the patient comprehends the concepts of CBT, follows through with the specific therapeutic exercises, understands the time-limited nature of CBT, and focuses on practical changes to overcoming barriers. Patients can be overwhelmed and regress if stressors come unexpectedly or arise in a multitude of situations, and if the therapeutic techniques used by the patient seem inadequate or not fully helpful. The patient must be made to understand that this is a normal part of treatment and, although CBT emphasizes the time limit of treatment, individual patient journeys can vary during this process. The therapist must validate the patient's feelings, and both parties need to work together in dealing with these issues.

Time Consciousness Remains the Key to Appropriate Cognitive Behavior Therapy Care

CBT therapy typically is short term, lasting for a few months, with the emphasis on patients' responses to a stressor and the way they can productively deal with them. Typically, patients can incorporate CBT techniques and use them effectively. Depending on the long-standing nature of a patient's mental health problems, CBT can last much longer. It is important that the roadmap of CBT initially involves a standard way of treating patients, with accommodations made to customize care. There are times when the roadmap might get jumbled and the patient may need acute care and admission for having suicidal thoughts, actively withdrawing from drugs or alcohol, or severe cognitive difficulties. The therapists must be aware of their limitations in the settings they find themselves in and be able to access care and resources as needed for the immediate well-being of their patients. There are often scenarios where a patient is under the treatment of both a psychiatrist and a CBT therapist and this combination might be the optimal treatment, especially if the patient also needs medication-based treatment. Using the diagnostic or symptomatic criteria based on the Diagnostic and Statistical Manual of Mental Disorders, Fifth Edition (DSM-55), this is considered the gold standard of care for some situations.[8]

Structured Practicality Remains a Bedrock of Cognitive Behavior Therapy

The structure remains important for patients who seek psychiatric care because exposure to unexpected stimuli is often one of the reasons patients decompensate mentally. CBT protocols emphasize this structure by:

1. Building initial rapport with the patient while discussing specific reasons the patient is at the office
2. Enlightening the patient about the prognosis and potential treatment regimens
3. Allowing patients to feel welcomed and able to communicate openly while validating their feelings
4. Explaining the time limitations of CBT therapy
5. Teaching the patient cognitive techniques to deal with a stressor while assisting the patient to embark on positive and helpful responses to the stressor
6. Having a plan in place in case the patient regresses

After the CBT treatment phase, future appointments, perhaps after a 3-month to 6-month period, allows therapists to monitor patients' successes and challenges in their mental health journeys. The therapists, on their part, must ensure that patients understand the techniques expected of them in dealing with stressors. Patients may need to voice these techniques back to ensure comprehension. It remains important for therapists to continuously elicit feedback on therapy sessions, patient comfort levels, patient-specific needs from the therapist, and homework completion monitoring, and for the therapist to provide feedback along with validation of the patient's feelings.[8]

Patients undergoing CBT are taught modalities on recognizing and screening self on their specific stressors and practicing techniques to challenge dysfunctional thoughts leading to negative outcomes.

The end goal of CBT is to assist patients in overcoming their anxiety, stress, or overwhelming feelings that can lead to negative outcomes when facing a stressor.[5] Most people are not able to corral their thoughts to their liking, allowing a multitude of unwelcome thoughts to intrude into a patient's mind. These thoughts can lead to self-doubt on the patient's part, leading to anxiety and depression. CBT techniques allow patients to put these thoughts to a test to screen their validity, a process taught by CBT practitioners and perfected by patients over time (eg, a patient thinking, "If I fail this test, I will never graduate, fail out of the university and be homeless, vs just comprehending that it is a stressor that just needs to be dealt with in a logical manner). CBT helps patients to monitor these automatic thoughts and screen them for logic and practicality. Patients are helped on this journey during treatment sessions. Role-play is a useful technique during these sessions to prepare patients for the expected stressors and how best to tackle them. The patients need to be made aware that they cannot fully control the thoughts they encounter, but they do have the power to deal with them in a productive and fulfilling manner. It stands to reason that patients in the throes of conditions such as depression and anxiety might view thoughts and stressors through a negative prism; therefore, these are scenarios that must be addressed by clinicians to help patients view them more realistically and pragmatically, a process that challenges these unrealistic assumptions.

Multiple Modalities of Cognitive Behavior Therapy Include Teaching Techniques to Mold Behavior and Changes in Thinking and Mood

CBT does have multiple subset iterations that may benefit specific patient populations or diagnostic conditions. These include:

- Cognitive processing therapy: a 12-week manualized therapy that has shown promise with patients with PTSD, especially after rape
- CT: short-term psychodynamic therapy often used in cases of anger management, bulimia, or obsessive-compulsive disorder (OCD)
- Dialectical behavior therapy: a specific type of cognitive psychotherapy that has shown potential improvement with borderline personality disorder, where the emphasis is on managing relationships and reducing interpersonal conflict[9]
- Rational emotive behavioral therapy: short-term psychotherapy that helps in reducing self-defeating thoughts and behaviors, allowing patients to initiate the process of empowering themselves

CBT therapists might involve aspects of different therapies to optimize care for their patients because some techniques might work better with certain conditions or people. Regardless, the fundamental concepts of CBT continue to revolve around dysfunctional thoughts, patient response to them, and cognitive strategies to overcome these negative emotions and actions.

Cognitive Behavior Therapy Indications for Usage

CBT is indicated in adults for anxiety disorders (panic disorder, agoraphobia, generalized anxiety disorder, social phobia), OCD, PTSD, IBS, chronic pain (eg, headaches, insomnia), personality disorders, and bulimia nervosa. CBT can also be an effective adjunctive treatment of patients with schizophrenia and bipolar disorder.[10]

In children and adolescents, CBT is indicated in the treatment of anxiety disorders, OCD, body dysmorphic disorder, PTSD, depression, tic disorders, Tourette syndrome, eating disorders, oppositional defiant disorder, chronic pain, and medical conditions (headaches, recurrent abdominal pain).[11] There is evidence to support efficacy in children and adolescents with high-functioning autism spectrum disorders.[12]

A CBT treatment course is typically weekly 30-minute to 1-hour sessions for a term of 9 to 15 weeks. The time range is influenced by the specific disorder or situation, the severity of symptoms, the chronicity of symptoms, the patient's progression, the patient's stress, and the patient's support system. The psychotherapist may be a psychiatrist, psychologist, licensed professional counselor, licensed social worker, licensed marriage and family therapist, psychiatric nurse, or any licensed professional with mental health training.[11] The therapist must meet state requirements for certification and licensure in the appropriate discipline and have expertise in treating the patient's particular complaints. The therapy is directed by the therapist and may be done for an individual patient, group, or family. CBT provides an active form of learning adaptive behavior and requires the therapist to provide the patient with information, skills, and the opportunity to develop adaptive coping mechanisms to change behavior.[13] The patient is an active participant, completing assignments as requested by the therapist. Each session is structured to meet specific predetermined goals, review assignments, and address new issues the patients may offer. To facilitate patient adaptability of learned coping skills and ensure success, the patient-provider relationship must be collaborative.[14] Patients must feel comfortable enough to let the provider know if concerns arise or the process is not meeting expectations. Because of the high patient compliance that is required for positive outcomes, the first detailed assessment of the patient's history, including social, occupational, relational, family, and assessment of social support, is essential before the start of therapy. Some of the common techniques taught and practiced in CBT are stress management, relaxation, resilience, assertiveness, and coping mechanisms.[12]

Patient Involvement and Education

Self-monitoring is a cognition technique helping patients become aware of the timing and occurrence of target symptoms to identify, assess, challenge thoughts, and apply strategies to improve their behavior.[15] Not all problems can be completely resolved. However, understanding the process of CBT provides a roadmap for patients to deal with stressors as they occur in future years. Educating patients about the CBT model empowers the patients to take part in their own progression and to set realistic treatment goals. Some benefit from reducing self-shame by normalizing aspects of their disorder. It is also a form of patient involvement that increases motivation and compliance. The ability to approach the therapy as a partnership with the therapist allows the opportunity to strengthen the relationship. CBT is most effective when the patient is an active participant and when decision making is shared. Once the short-term therapy is complete, patients ideally should use learned skills to recognize early signs of a relapse in symptoms.[16] Future sessions may be necessary to review the skills learned throughout the therapy.

SUMMARY

At the current time, CBT dominates psychotherapy as the most widely validated first-line treatment option in a multitude of psychosocial pathologic disorders such as anxiety, depression, personality disorders, and addiction treatment. Although proved to be efficacious, there is room for further improvement because trials suggest significant rates of patient dropout and/or relapse. Newer areas of psychotherapy are dialectical behavior therapy for the treatment of borderline personality disorder and acceptance and commitment therapy.[16] Using these new concepts in a multidimensional approach along with traditional cognitive and behavioral principles for the treatment of complex disorders, especially those with high relapse rates, may open the door to significant positive mental health outcomes and an improved understanding of mental disorder.

CLINICS CARE POINTS

- CBT is a short-term form of psychotherapy
- CBT empowers patients to change dysfunctional types of thinking that lead to negative outcomes
- CBT must be practiced with mutual respect and transparency between patient and therapist
- CBT includes homework assignments for the patient, and feedback from the patient is critical in moving forward with therapy
- CBT involves validation of the patient's feelings by the therapist
- CBT has been proved to be effective in treatment of major depression and anxiety disorders

ACKNOWLEDGMENTS

None.

REFERENCES

1. Drake K, Keeton CP, Ginsburg GS. Cognitive Behavioral Therapy (CBT): Johns Hopkins Psychiatry Guide. Cognitive Behavioral Therapy (CBT) | Johns Hopkins Psychiatry Guide. 2020. Available at: https://www.hopkinsguides.com/hopkins/view/Johns_Hopkins_Psychiatry_Guide/787145/all/Cognitive_Behavioral_Therapy__CBT_. Accessed August 31, 2020.
2. Cherry K. Albert Ellis' influence on the field of psychology. Verywell Mind 2007. Available at: https://www.verywellmind.com/albert-ellis-biography-2795493. Accessed August 31, 2020.
3. Cognitive therapy: current Status and future Directions. Available at: https://www.annualreviews.org/doi/abs/10.1146/annurev-med-052209-100032.   Accessed August 31, 2020.
4. Sprinch SE, Olatunji BO, Reese HE, et al. Cognitive-behavioral therapy, behavioral therapy, and cognitive therapy. In: Beck J, editor. Massachusetts general hospital: comprehensive clinical psychiatry. 2nd edition. London: Elsevier; 2016. p. 152–63.
5. Beck JS. Cognitive therapy: Basics and beyond. New York: Guilford Press; 2011.
6. Carpenter JK, Andrews LA, Witcraft SM, et al. Cognitive-behavioral therapy for anxiety and related disorders: A meta-analysis of randomized placebo-controlled trials. Depress Anxiety 2018;35:502–14.
7. Leichsenring F, Steinert C. Is cognitive-behavioral therapy the gold standard for psychotherapy? The need for plurality in treatment and research. JAMA 2017; 318(14):1323–4.
8. Grohol JM. CPT Codes for psychology Services. Psych central 2018. Available at: https://psychcentral.com/lib/cpt-codes-for-psychology-services/. Accessed August 31, 2020.
9. David D, Cotet C, Matu S, et al. 50 years of rational-emotive and cognitive-behavioral therapy: A systematic review and meta-analysis. J Clin Psychol 2018;74: 304–18.
10. Liness S, Beale S, Lea S, et al. Evaluating CBT clinical competence with standardised role plays and patient therapy sessions. Cogn Ther Res 2019;43(6): 959–70.
11. Hayes SC, Hofmann SG. The third wave of cognitive-behavioral therapy and the rise of process-based care. World Psychiatry 2017;16(3):245–6.
12. Walter HJ, DeMaso DR. Psychotherapy and psychiatric hospitalization. In: Beck J, editor. Nelson textbook of pediatrics. 21st edition. Philadelphia: Elsevier Inc; 2020. p. 197–201.
13. Murphy A, Bourke J, Flynn D, et al. A cost-effectiveness analysis of dialectical behavior therapy for treating individuals with borderline personality disorder in the community. Ir J Med Sci 2020;189(2):415–23.
14. Duarte R, Lloyd A, Kotas E, et al. Are acceptance and mindfulness-based interventions 'value for money'? Evidence from a systematic literature review. Br J Clin Psychol 2019;58(2):187–210.
15. Karyotaki E, Riper H, Twisk J, et al. Efficacy of self-guided internet-based cognitive behavioral therapy in the treatment of depressive symptoms: a meta-analysis of individual participant data. JAMA Psychiatry 2017;74(4):351–9.
16. Walter HJ, Bukstein OG, Abright AR, et al. Clinical Practice Guideline for the Assessment and Treatment of Children and Adolescents with Anxiety Disorders. J Am Acad Child Adolesc Psychiatry 2020;8–9. https://doi.org/10.1016/j.jaac.2020.05.005.

It's all About the Meds
Understanding the Principles of Psychopharmacotherapy

Samantha Salyer, PharmD, MS Ed[a,b,*]

KEYWORDS

- Pharmacodynamics • Pharmacokinetics • Comorbidities • Drug-drug interactions
- Pharmacotherapy • Elderly

KEY POINTS

- Many drug-drug interactions exist.
- Elderly populations are at increased risk of adverse effects.
- Many agents have multiple uses.
- Drug dosages range can vary greatly between patients.
- Always use the minimum effective dose.

INTRODUCTION

In recent years, the number of psychotropic medications on the market has increased drastically as has the number of psychotropic prescriptions.[1,2] Primary care clinicians write 65% of all psychotropic medication prescriptions and 80% of all anxiolytic and antidepressant prescriptions.[1,2] With this increase in prescribing rates, along with the increase in the number of providers prescribing psychotropic medications, the likelihood of drug interactions occurring is high. Drug-drug interactions are associated with a higher risk of hospitalization rates, treatment failure, avoidable medical complications, patient death, and increased overall health care costs.[2] Many patients with psychiatric conditions will have significant comorbidities including cardiovascular disease, diabetes, chronic obstructive pulmonary disease, and/or chronic pain.[3] In recent years, interdisciplinary collaboration has shifted from a model to reality. With collaboration of different health care professions, patients can get better care and improved health outcomes.[4]

[a] Emory & Henry College, School of Health Sciences, 565 Radio Hill Road, Marion, VA 24354, USA; [b] Walgreens Company
* Emory & Henry College, School of Health Sciences, 565 Radio Hill Road, Marion, VA 24354.
E-mail address: ssalyer@ehc.edu

Physician Assist Clin 6 (2021) 381–394
https://doi.org/10.1016/j.cpha.2021.02.003
2405-7991/21/© 2021 Elsevier Inc. All rights reserved.

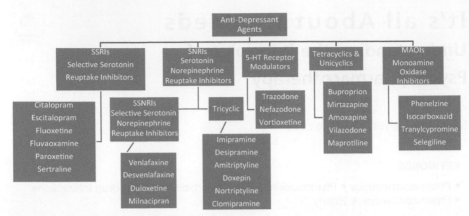

Fig. 1. Pharmacotherapy in behavioral medicine.

SELECTIVE SEROTONIN REUPTAKE INHIBITORS

Selective serotonin reuptake inhibitors (SSRIs) **(Fig. 1)** are a widely prescribed class of medications with a tolerable adverse effect profile and low cost; they are also deemed relatively safe **(Table 1)**. Their use is further boosted by the broad spectrum of conditions that can be treated: generalized anxiety, post-traumatic stress disorder, bulimia, obsessive-compulsive disorder, panic disorder, and postmenstrual dysphoric disorder.[5] SSRIs are considered first-line treatments in depression disorders.[6] These medications work by blocking the serotonin transporter. Dosage ranges vary depending on the condition being treated and patient response.

As a class, SSRIs can increase serotonergic activity throughout the body, resulting in gastrointestinal (GI) discomfort and sexual dysfunction. SSRIs can also cause headache, weight gain and lead to insomnia. Fluoxetine is considered an activating medication and must be given in the morning to decrease the incidence of insomnia. Weight gain tends to occur more with paroxetine. All SSRIs carry a risk of birth defects if taken during pregnant; paroxetine is associated with the highest risk. Elderly (65 or greater) patients should be started at the lowest dose available to prevent unwanted adverse effects.[7]

Sudden withdrawal of an SSRI can lead to a withdrawal or discontinuation syndrome. This is most prevalent with the shorter-acting forms of SSRIs and most likely to occur after a patient has been taking an antidepressant for at least 6 weeks. Symptoms of discontinuation syndrome include dizziness, nausea, hyperarousal (anxiety and agitation), influenzalike symptoms, insomnia and/or sensory disturbances. Symptoms are generally mild and should subside within about 2 weeks of discontinuation or sooner if a second agent is started.[8]

Serotonin syndrome is a serious effect seen in patients who take multiple medications that affect serotonin levels. Improper drug-drug combinations are often the cause of serotonin syndrome. Patients will present with various complaints: hyperthermia, hypertension, diarrhea, mydriasis, tremor, agitation, and coma in severe cases.[5] Unlike neuroleptic malignant syndrome, onset in serotonin syndrome usually occurs quickly (within a few hours). Serotonin syndrome can occur with the first dose of a serotonergic drug, but is more likely to occur when multiple offending agents are given together. In combination with SSRIs, commonly used drugs such as ondansetron, tramadol, triptans (class of migraine medications), fentanyl, and selective serotonin norepinephrine reuptake inhibitors (SSNRIs) can cause serotonin syndrome.

Table 1
Selective serotonin reuptake inhibitors[5,6,9,10]

Drug (Generic)	Drug (Brand)	Dose Range	Usual Dose
Fluoxetine	Prozac	10–80 mg	20 mg
Fluoxetine (once weekly)	Prozac	90 mg	90 mg
Paroxetine	Paxil	10–60 mg	20 mg
Paroxetine CR (controlled release)	Paxil CR	12.5–75 mg	25 mg
Fluvoxamine	Luvox	50–300 mg	50 mg
Sertraline	Zoloft	25–200 mg	50 mg
Citalopram	Celexa	10–40 mg	20 mg
Escitalopram	Lexapro	5–20 mg	10 mg

Ondansetron and triptan agents are used frequently with SSRIs and normally do not precipitate serotonin syndrome as they are used for a limited time. Less frequently used drugs that can be linked to serotonin syndrome include: monoamine oxidase inhibitors (MAOIs), linezolid, meperidine, and herbals (eg, St. John's Wort and ginseng).[5,9,10]

SEROTONIN NOREPINEPHRINE REUPTAKE INHIBITORS

SSNRI's and tricyclic antidepressants (TCAs) both have similar actions but are not structurally related (**Table 2**). Both classes bind to the serotonin transporter and the norepinephrine transporter with varying selectivity. TCAs have decreased in use because of the development of newer, much safer alternatives. Tricyclics have an increased risk of overdose that can be worrisome in patients with psychological disorders. There is also an increased risk of prolonging the QT interval.

SSNRIs are more likely to cause noradrenergic effects, which can increase blood pressure and heart rate, than the SSRIs.[5] Some central nervous system (CNS) activation can present as agitation, insomnia and/or anxiety. Immediate-release venlafaxine is most likely to cause adverse effects.[5] Duloxetine can potentially damage the liver. All drugs in this class can cause discontinuation syndrome if abruptly stopped or not properly tapered.

Table 2
Selective serotonin-norepinephrine reuptake inhibitors[5,6,9,10]

Drug(Generic)	Drug (Brand)	Dose Range	Usual Dose
Venlafaxine	Effexor	75–225 mg Up to 375 mg (inpatient only)	75–150 mg
Venlafaxine ER (extended release)	Effexor XR	75–225 mg	75–150 mg
Desvenlafaxine	Pristiq	25–400 mg	50–400 mg
Duloxetine	Cymbalta	20–120 mg	30–60 mg
Milnacipran[a]	Savella	12.5–200 mg	25–50 mg
Levomilnacipran	Fetzima	20–120 mg	40–120 mg

[a] Currently no indication for depression only indicated for fibromyalgia in the United States.

Tricyclic antidepressants have fallen out of favor for use in depression (**Table 3**). This is attributed to risk of overdose and the anticholinergic effects that can be seen with their use. Patients often complain of dry mouth, dry eyes, urinary retention, and constipation with tricyclics. For the most part, these agents are reserved for use for treatment-resistant individuals and are often used off-label for other indications (restless legs, insomnia, or migraine prevention).[5]

5-HT RECEPTOR MODULATORS

Serotonin (5-HT) receptor modulators are a group of medications that work as antagonists at serotonin receptor sites (**Table 4**). All 3 medications are inhibitors of serotonin transporter. Nefazodone has a weak inhibitory effect on the norepinephrine transporter. Nefazodone has a US Food and Drug Administration (FDA) black box warning linking it to hepatotoxicity that can be lethal. Because of this warning, nefazodone is not commonly prescribed. Both nefazodone and trazodone are labeled for use in depression but also possess a sedative effect that can work well for patients with issues of insomnia. All SRMs can cause GI discomfort (nausea and vomiting). There are limited instances where trazodone can cause priapism. Vortioxetine is only available as a brand name medication and has limited use because of cost. However, it is frequently used in the outpatient setting for its effectiveness in depression with limited adverse effects. GI discomfort and sexual dysfunction are most common adverse effects and occur more frequently with higher doses.[5]

Table 3
Tricyclic antidepressants[5,6,9,10]

Drug (Generic)	Drug (Brand)	Dose Range	Usual Dose
Imipramine	Tofranil	50–200 mg Up to 300 mg (inpatient only)	50–150 mg
Imipramine	Tofranil PM	75–200 mg Up to 300 mg (inpatient only)	75–150 mg
Desipramine	Norpramin	50–300 mg	100–200 mg
Amitrityline	Elavil	40–150 mg Up to 300 mg (inpatient only)	50–100 mg
Doxepin	Sinequan	25–300 mg	75–150 mg
Nortriptyline	Pamelor	10–150 mg	50–150 mg
Clomipramine	Anafranil	25–250 mg	100–200 mg

TETRACYCLICS AND UNICYCLICS

Bupropion has a unique unicyclic aminoketone structure. Bupropion and its active metabolite appear to be inhibitors of norepinephrine and dopamine reuptake. They also have a more definitive effect on presynaptic levels of norepinephrine and dopamine. Bupropion resembles amphetamine in its chemical structure and acts as an activating drug.[5] Because of this, it should be dosed in the morning. Mirtazapine and amoxapine are similar to TCAs and possess some anticholinergic properties. Both drugs are inhibitors of the norepinephrine transporter and show mild activity as serotonin transporter inhibitors. Amoxapine shows some inhibitory effects on dopamine

Table 4
5-HT receptor modulators[5,6,9,10]

Drug (Generic)	Drug (Brand)	Dose Range	Usual Dose
Nefazodone	Serzone	50–600 mg	300–600 mg
Trazodone	Desyrel	50–400 mg Up to 600 mg (inpatient only)	150–300 mg
Vortioxetine	Trintellix[a]	5–20 mg	20 mg

[a] Formerly known as Brintellix.

receptors, thus giving it antipsychotic properties. Vilazodone works in a variety of ways by acting as a serotonin reuptake inhibitor and as a partial agonist of serotonin receptors. Because of this action, it also has some activity as an antianxiety medication. Starting doses can differ between patients and formulations chosen, but target doses are generally with in a determined range (**Table 5**).

Table 5
Tetracyclics and unicyclics[5,6,9,10]

Drug (Generic)	Drug (Brand)	Dose Range	Usual Dose
Bupropion IR[a]	Wellbutrin	75–450 mg	200–300 mg
SR/ER (12 h)		100–400 mg	100–200 mg
ER/XL (24 h)		150–450 mg	150–300 mg
Mirtazapine[b]	Remeron	7.5–45 mg	15–45 mg
Amoxapine	Asendin	25–400 mg Up to 600 mg (inpatient only)	200–400 mg
Maprotiline	Ludiomil	25–225 mg	75–150 mg
Vilazodone	Viibryd	10–40 mg	20–40 mg

[a] Bupropion IR single doses should not exceed 150 mg; all forms should be titrated up/down slowly because of the risk of seizures.[9]
[b] Available as an ODT (orally disintegrating tablet).

MAOIS

MAOIs were the first class of medications developed to treat depression. As a class, they are limited in their use because of toxicities and the number of drug/food interactions that can occur. In practice, MAOIs are prescribed for patients who have not responded to other medications. Phenelzine, isocarboxazid, and tranylcypromine all irreversibly bind with monoamine oxidase A and B. Selegiline is more selective in its binding and is mostly an irreversible inhibitor of monoamine oxidase B and at higher doses does exhibit inhibition of monoamine oxidase A. Selegiline is dispensed in Parkinson disease as a capsule, tablet or ODT. It is also available in the patch form for treatment of depression. MAOIs or their metabolites resemble amphetamines by producing stimulating effects on the CNS. MAOIs all experience high first-pass metabolism rates and will inhibit monoamine oxidase in the gut. This property causes a

Table 6
Foods to avoid with monoamine oxidase inhibitors[6,9,10]

Aged Cheeses	Broad beans or pods (Fava Beans)	Licorice
Air Dried Meats	Soy sauce	Canned or processed meats
Cured/Smoked Meats	Marmite	Snails
Beer	Raisins	Fermented foods
Herring	Canned Figs	Liver
Sardines	Ripe Avocado	Yeast extract or products
Anchovies	Sauerkraut	Caffeine containing foods/drinks
Sour cream	Yogurt/Cottage Cheese	Wine
Pickled Meats	Raspberries	Bananas

*Can have a single glass of white wine or cocktail; up to 56 grams of caffeine per day is acceptable; up to 56 grams of yogurt/cottage cheese/sour cream is allowed per day.[6,10]

Table 7
Medications to avoid with monoamine oxidase inhibitors[6,9,10]

Amephetamines	Decongestants	Dextromethorphan	Levodopa
Meperidine	Methyldopa	Methylphenidate	Antidepressants[a]
Other MAOI's	Triptans (Migraine HA)	Tolcapone/Entacapone	Reserpine
Carbamazepine	Cocaine	Cyclobenzaprine	Chlorthalidone
Oxcarbazipine	Propofol	Ketamine	Clonidine
Codeine	St. Johns Wart	Methylene Blue	Morphine
Procarbazine	Sympathomimetics	Tramadol	Yohimbine

[a] Not TCAs (tricyclic antidepressants); HA (headache); MAOIs (monoamine oxidase inhibitors).

Table 8
Monoamine oxidase inhibitors[5,6,9,10]

Drug (Generic)	Drug (Brand)	Dose Range	Usual Dose
Phenelzine	Nardil	15–90 mg	45–60 mg
Isocarboxazid	Marplan	10–60 mg	20–60 mg
Tranylcypromine	Parnate	10–60 mg	30–60 mg
Selegiline	Emsam	6–12 mg	6–12 mg

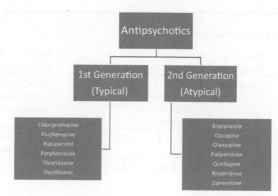

Fig. 2. Antipsychotics.

high number of food interactions (**Table 6**). MAOIs have a high incidence of sexual dysfunction and drug interactions, including over-the-counter medications. (**Table 7**). Common adverse reactions include orthostatic hypotension, weight gain, insomnia, or restlessness. Phenelzine does not cause CNS activation, instead causing sedation. Confusion can be seen at higher doses, and sudden discontinuation syndrome can occur with a delirium-like presentation. When starting a patient on these medications, start at the lowest dose and increase until the desired effect occurs within the target range or adverse effects become intolerable for the patient (**Table 8**).

FIRST-GENERATION ANTIPSYCHOTIC AGENTS (TYPICAL)

All antipsychotic agents (**Fig. 2**) block dopamine D_2 receptors, and most block the serotonin 5-HT$_{2A}$ receptors to varying degrees. The higher the blockade, the higher the adverse effect profile seen. As a category of medications, most typical antipsychotic agents produce extrapyramidal adverse effects as dose escalation occurs. Extrapyramidal adverse effects include dystonia, akathisia, pseudoparkinsonism and/or tardive dyskinesia. First-generation agents are more likely to cause hyperprolactinemia than second-generation agents. Both generations of antipsychotic medications have the potential to cause neuroleptic malignant syndrome (NMS); however, fluphenazine and haloperidol seem to be the most likely to cause the reaction.[9,10] Patients will typically present within 1 to 3 days with acute onset of parkinsonism, hyperthermia, and hypertension.[5] Sedation can occur with all agents but is likely to be more severe with chlorpromazine and thioridazine. Fluphenazine and haloperidol are both available as a longer-acting deconate form. Each agent has specific dosing ranges that can differ based on patient response (**Table 9**).

SECOND-GENERATION ANTIPSYCHOTIC AGENTS (ATYPICAL)

This group of medications has a more tolerable adverse effect profile and fewer drug interactions. Most medications in the category of atypical antipsychotics (see **Fig. 2**) have a greater affinity to affect 5-HT$_{2A}$ receptors and limited dopamine D_2 receptor interaction. Because of less affinity for D_2 receptors, atypical agents are less likely to cause extrapyramidal adverse effects than first-generation antipsychotics. Clozapine has strict guidelines for prescribing and dispensing. Patients have to have blood work to monitor for agranulocytosis, and the absolute neutrophil counts (ANCs) have

Table 9
Antipsychotic agents (1st generation)[5,6,9,10]

Drug (Generic)[a]	Drug (Brand)	Dosage Range	Usual Dose	Specific Adverse Effects/Special Notes
Chlorpromazine	Thorazine	100–1000 mg Up to 2000 mg (short-term inpatient)	30–1000 mg[b]	Sedation, orthostatic hypotension, anticholinergic effects
Fluphenazine (oral)	Prolixin	2.5–40 mg	2.5–20 mg	Neuroleptic malignant syndrome (NMS)
Fluphenazine IM (immediate-release)	Prolixin	1.25–10 mg	2.5–10 mg	
Fluphenazine Deconate	Prolixin Deconate	6.25–25 mg	6.25 mg-25 mg	
Haloperidol (oral)	Haldol	1.5–20 mg	Acute 6–20 mg Maintenance 6–12 mg	Higher dose may be needed for refractory patients; NMS possible
Haloperidol lactate (intramuscular)	Haldol IM	2–20 mg	2–20 mg	Dosed every 4–6 h
Haloperidol deconate	Haldol Dec	50–450 mg	50–200 mg	Initial dose should not exceed 100 mg; patients should be stabilized on an immediate-release formulation before initiation; dosed every 4 weeks
Perphenazine	Trilafon	8–24 mg Up to 64 mg (short term)	12–24 mg	
Thioridazine	Mellaril	50–800 mg	200–800 mg	Sedation, orthostatic hypotension, anticholinergic effects, Life-threatening arrhythmias
Thiothixene	Navane	2–60 mg	20–30 mg	

[a] Common first-generation adverse effect—EPS and hyperprolactinemia.
[b] Range depends on severity of presentation; intramuscular (IM) injection may be required.

to be 500/mm^3 or above.[10] Both aripiprazole and risperidone have sustained-released formulations that can be dosed monthly. Dosing varies depending on formulation used and patient response (**Table 10**).

MOOD STABILIZERS

Mood stabilizers (**Fig. 3**) are frequently prescribed in patients with bipolar disorder. Some atypical and antidepressants have efficacy in specific phases of bipolar disorder and are approved treatment options. Lithium has been a mainstream treatment for many years; however, some providers are choosing newer antipsychotics for treatment. Lithium acts by normalizing second messenger systems and increasing serotonin levels. Much of lithium's actions are not fully understood, but the medication can take 5 days to reach a steady state and has a narrow therapeutic window,

Table 10
Second-generation agents (atypical)[5,6,9,10]

Drug (Generic)	Drug (Brand)	Dosage Range	Usual Dose	Specific Adverse Effects/ Special Notes
Aripiprazole (oral)	Abilify	2–30 mg	10–30 mg	Drowsiness is common
Aripiprazole (extended release) ER injection	Abilify Maintena	300–400 mg	300 mg	Initial dose is usually 400 mg with oral form for 14 d; maintenance dose 300 mg
Aripiprazole lauroxil ER injection	Aristada	441–882 mg	441–882 mg	First dose given with oral aripiprazole
Clozapine	Clozaril	12.5–900 mg	300–600 mg	Anticholinergic, agranulocytosis, diabetes, hypercholesterolemia, orthostatic hypotension, sedation, weight gain
Olanzapine (oral)	Zyprexa	5–20 mg	10–20 mg	Diabetes, hypercholesterolemia, weight gain
Olanzapine (IM)	Zyprexa IM	2.5–30 mg	5–10 mg	Improvement seen within 15–30 min; initial dose for agitation 10 mg
Quetiapine	Seroquel	25–800 mg	150–800 mg	Moderate sedation
Quetiapine ER	Seroquel XR	50–800 mg	300–800 mg	Moderate sedation; most patients require 300–400 mg/d
Risperidone	Risperdal	1–16 mg	4–16	Hyperprolactinemia
Ziprasidone	Geodon	20–160 mg	80–160	QT prolongation; food increases bioavailability

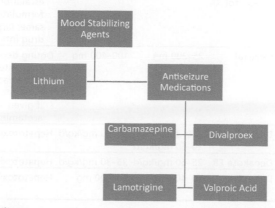

Fig. 3. Mood stabilizers.

requiring frequent serum monitoring. Serum levels should be checked on day 3 of treatment, 10 to 12 hours after the last dose.[5,9] Patients with acute mania need a therapeutic blood level of 0.8 to 1.2 mEq/L and a maintenance blood level of 0.8 to 1 mEq/L.[9] Some patients can be maintained at lower levels, but that is uncommon.[5] No true maximum dose limitation has been set for lithium; however serum levels of 1.5 mEq/L or greater should be avoided because of adverse effects and toxicities (especially kidney).[9] Lamotrigine, carbamazepine, and valprioic acid are all classified as antiseizure medications. Lamotrigine has to be tapered over time, and the tapering schedule depends on whether it is coadministered with carbamazepine or valproate or dosed alone. Dosing depends on patient response and tolerability (**Table 11**).

DRUG-DRUG INTERACTIONS

The combination of anticholinergic and antipsychotic agents will increase the occurrence and severity of anticholinergic adverse effects (dry eyes, urinary retention, and constipation). Commonly used anticholinergic agents include atropine, dicyclomine, hyoscyamine, and scopolamine. A synergistic effect can be seen when sedative drugs are added to antipsychotic drugs. Medications that would potentiate this effect include other antipsychotics, sedatives, hypnotics, melatonin, diphenhydramine, and

Table 11
Mood-stabilizing agents[5,6,9,10]

Drug (Generic)	Drug Brand	Dosage Range	Usual Dose	Special Adverse Effects/Notes
Lithium (IM)	Eskalith	300–1800 mg	1200–1800 mg	Monitor for blood levels at day 3 12 hours after last dose
Lithium (ER)	Eskalith CR; Lithobid	450–1200 mg	900–1200 mg	Dosing has to be in multiples of 450 in divided doses; if uneven dosing occurs, give highest in the evening
Antiseizure Drugs/Mood-Stabilizing Agents				
Carbamazepine (IR/ER)	Tegretol/ Tegretol XR	200–1800 mg	600–1600 mg	Ranges for dosing and escalation for XR and IR formulations are the same; large number of drug interactions
Lamotrigine	Lamictal	25–200 mg	100–400 mg	Dosing depends on use of valproate/ carbamazepine; hepatotoxicity can occur if given with acetaminophen
Divalproex delayed release	Depakote	750–3000 mg 20–60 mg/kg/d	20–30 mg/kg/d	Hepatotoxic
Divalproex ER	Depakote ER	25–60 mg/kg/d	25–30 mg/kg/d	Hepatotoxic
Valproic acid/ valproate	Depakene	50–400 mg	50–400 mg	Hepatotoxic

Abbreviations: CR, controlled release; ER/XR, extended release.

Table 12
Drug-drug interactions for antipsychotic agents[5,6,9–12]

Antipsychotic Agent	Increase Metabolism (Less of the Agent in the Blood Stream)	Decrease Metabolism (More of the Agent in the Blood Stream)		Enzyme System Involved
Aripiprazole	Carbamazepine Oxcarbazepine Phenobarbital Phenytoin Rifampin Glucocorticoids Modafinil St. John's Wort	Bupropion Duloxetine Fluoxetine Fluvoxamine Paroxetine Sertraline Indinavir Nelfinavir Ritonavir Clarithromycin Erythromycin Fluconazole Ketoconazole	Itraconazole Chlorpheniramine Diltiazem Quinidine Diphenhydramine Cimetidine Grapefruit Haloperidol Hydroxyzine Verapamil	CYP2D6 CYP3A4
Clozapine	Carbamazepine Phenobarbital Phenytoin Rifampin Glucocorticoids Modafinil St. John's Wort	Fluoxetine Fluvoxamine Indinavir Nelfinavir Ritonavir Clarithromycin Erythromycin Fluconazole Ketoconazole	Itraconazole Diltiazem Cimetidine Grapefruit Haloperidol Omeprazole Ticlopidine Topiramate Verapamil	CYP3A4 CYP1A2 CYP2C19
Haloperidol	Carbamazepine Oxcarbazepine Phenobarbital Phenytoin Rifampin St John's Wort Tobacco Glucocorticoids Insulin products Modafinil Omeprazole	Bupropion Duloxetine Fluoxetine Fluvoxamine Paroxetine Sertraline Indinavir Nelfinavir Ritonavir Clarithromycin Erythromycin Fluconazole	Fluoroquinolones Ketoconazole Itraconazole Chlorpheniramine Diltiazem Quinidine Diphenhydramine Cimetidine Grapefruit Hydroxyzine Verapamil	CYP2D6 CYP3A4 CYP1A2
Olanzapine Quetiapine	Carbamazepine Oxcarbazepine Phenobarbital Phenytoin Rifampin Glucocorticoids Modafinil Omeprazole St Johns Wart Nicotine (Olanzapine only)	Fluvoxamine Indinavir Nelfinavir Ritonavir Clarithromycin Erythromycin Fluconazole Ketoconazole	Itraconazole Diltiazem Cimetidine Grapefruit Verapamil Fluoroquinolones (Olanzapine only)	CYP3A4 (Both drugs CYP1A2 (Olanzapine only)

(continued on next page)

Table 12 (continued)			
Antipsychotic Agent	Increase Metabolism (Less of the Agent in the Blood Stream)	Decrease Metabolism (More of the Agent in the Blood Stream)		Enzyme System Involved
Risperidone	Dexamethasone Rifampin	Bupropion Duloxetine Fluoxetine Paroxetine Cimetidine	Quinidine Chlorpheniramine Diphenhydramine Haloperidol Hydroxyzine	CYP2D6

tricyclic antidepressants (**Table 12**). Enzyme induction and inhibition have a profound effect on drug concentrations. The main enzymes that are involved are CYP2D6, CYP3A4, CYP1A2, CYP2C19.[6]

SEIZURE DISORDERS

Patients with psychiatric diagnoses often have seizure disorders.[12] Many psychotropic medications can be associated with a lower seizure threshold. Because of this interaction, the frequency and severity of seizures increase. Many patients with seizure disorders also have comorbid psychiatric conditions: depression, anxiety, personality disorders, and/or psychosis.[11,12] As a class, antidepressants carry a low risk of inducing seizures. In the antidepressant class, amoxapine, clomipramine, and maprotiline have the highest incidence of inducing seizures. All 3 medications should be avoided in patients with epilepsy.[12] Patients who ingest toxic levels of desipramine, imipramine, or nortriptyline have a high risk of seizures. SSRIs and SNRIs are preferred treatment options for patients with seizure disorders. Bupropion IR carries a high risk of seizures and is contraindicated in these patients.[11] The SR and XL formulations carry a lower risk of seizure activity. MAOIs have a low seizure risk but do have a high incidence of serotonin syndrome associated with their use. First-generation antipsychotic agents are associated with seizure activity. Of these agents, chlorpromazine and loxapine are associated with the highest risk.[12] Atypical antipsychotics (second generation) also carry a risk of seizure activity. Clozapine was associated with a risk of seizure, as doses increase to 600 mg/d. Ziprasidone, aripiprazole, and risperidone have been shown to have no significant risk of seizure activity.[12]

CONSIDERATIONS FOR THE ELDERLY

The elderly population is increasing in the United States, with medication dosing a growing concern because of adverse effects and drug-drug interactions seen with a large number of antidepressants and antipsychotics. Elderly patients typically present with comorbid conditions. Elderly patients often present with a higher incidence of hypertension, diabetes, hyperlipidemia, and/or kidney dysfunction. It is extremely important to know the medications that are contraindicated in the older patient or in the patient with comorbidities.

In general, antidepressants that should be avoided in elderly patients include amitriptyline, amoxapine, clomipramine, doxepin, imipramine, nortriptyline, paroxetine, protriptyline and trimipramine (**Table 13**).[13] This group of medications has

Table 13 Medications to avoid in the elderly[13]	
Amitriptyline	Imipramine
Amoxapine	Nortriptyline
Clomipramine	Paroxetine
Doxepin (doses >6 mg/d)	Protriptyline Trimipramine
1st Generation Antipsychotics	2nd Generation Antipsychotics

anticholinergic adverse effects that can be dangerous for the elderly. Adverse effects such as orthostatic hypotension or sedation can lead to falls and injuries that can be life threatening or life altering. Other adverse effects of the anticholinergics such as dry mouth, urinary retention, decreased ability to sweat, constipation, and/or dry eyes are less life altering but often concerning to the patient.

Antipsychotics of either generation should be avoided in elderly patients. When antipsychotics are given to elderly patients, they can increase the risk of cerebrovascular accidents. They can also increase the risk of cognitive decline, thereby increasing mortality in dementia patients.[13] Antipsychotics should not be considered a mainstream treatment for behavioral issues associated with dementia or delirium. Antipsychotics are considered a later treatment option and only if non-pharmacological treatments have failed or patients might potentially harm themselves or others. Antipsychotic agents may be used in elderly patients presenting with schizophrenia or bipolar disorder, with the risk outweighing the chance of harm.[13]

SUMMARY

Overall, there are many medications to choose from when treating a mental health patient. Care for mental health patients is often chronic, if not lifelong, which means patients will likely develop comorbidities. It is important to consider age of the patient along with known comorbidities when choosing a treatment medication. Adverse effects are likely to occur no matter which medication is chosen, but most usually dissipate over time. Providers should choose a drug with tolerable adverse effects and limited or no drug interactions for patients, as much as possible. New therapies and recommendations are constantly evolving for mental health patients, so it is important to utilize all resources available including the multidisciplinary team. Teams of providers provide the best outcomes for patients by sharing their expertise.

DISCLOSURE

The author has no conflict of interest or relationship with any drug manufacturer mentioned in the article. No financial relationship exists with any commercial company with direct financial interest in subject matter presented.

REFERENCES

1. English BA, Dortch M, Ereshefsky L, et al. Clinically significant psychotropic drug-drug interactions in the primary care setting. Curr Psychiatry Rep 2012; 14(4):376–90.
2. Lieberman JA. The use of antipsychotics in primary care. J Clin Psychiatry 2003; 5(Suppl 3):3–8.

3. Alderman CP, Lucca JM. Psychiatry and clinical pharmacy: a logical partnership. Indian J Psychiatry 2017;59(2):138–40.
4. Keltner NL, Moore RL. Biological perspectives psychiatric drug-drug interactions: a review. Perspect Psychiatr Care 2010;46(3):244–51.
5. Katzong B, Trevor A. Basic and clinical pharmacology. New York: McGraw Hill; 2015.
6. Dipiro J, Talbert R, Yee G, et al. Pharmacotherapy: a pathophysiologic approach. New York: McGraw Hill; 2008.
7. Laatikainen O, Sneck S, Bloigu R, et al. Hospitalizations due to adverse drug events in the elderly-a retrospective register study. Front Pharmacol 2016;7:358.
8. Warner CH, Bobo W, Warner C, et al. Antidepressant discontinuation syndrome. Am Fam Physician 2006;74(3):449–56.
9. Clinical Pharmacology [Internet]. Tampa (FL): Elsevier. c2020. Available at: http://www.clinicalpharmacology.com. Accessed July 15, 2020.
10. Access Medicine (internet). New York: McGraw Hill. C2020. Available at: accessmedicine.mhmedical.com. Accessed July 1, 2020.
11. Monaco F, Cicolin A. Interactions between anticonvulsant and psychoactive drugs. Epilepsia 1999;40(Suppl 10):S71–6.
12. Habibi M, Hart F, Bainbridge J. The impact of psychoactive drugs on seizures and antiepileptic drugs. Curr Neurol Neurosci Rep 2016;16(8):71.
13. 2019 American Geriatrics Society Beers Criteria® Update Expert Panel. American Geriatrics Society 2019 updated AGS beers criteria for potentially inappropriate medication use in older adults. J Am Geriatr Soc 2019;67(4):674–94.

It's Not About the Meds

Understanding the Principles of Nonpharmacologic Interventions in the Treatment of Depression

Nicole E. Miller, PA-C

KEYWORDS

- Electroconvulsive therapy • Transcranial magnetic stimulation • Depression
- Adjunctive therapy • Nonpharmacologic • Psychotherapy

KEY POINTS

- Pharmacotherapy should almost never be used as monotherapy.
- Nonpharmacologic intervention in addition to pharmacotherapy is more beneficial in alleviating depressive symptoms than medication alone.
- Electroconvulsive therapy is the gold standard treatment of refractory depression.

INTRODUCTION

Modern-day medications have had a positive impact in treating depression and other mental illnesses. Serotonin and norepinephrine modulators are beneficial in improving symptoms and the overall quality of life for individuals diagnosed with depression, anxiety, or other psychiatric disorders. Although medications can have many positive effects on the symptoms of depression, they can also cause adverse side effects, such as nausea, insomnia, anxiety, and even sexual dysfunction.[1] These adverse effects may deter patients from taking medications or cause patients to discontinue medications on their own.[2] There are several nonpharmacologic techniques, procedures, and lifestyle changes that can be used to augment treatment outcomes in conjunction with medications. These techniques can be used to reduce the need for additional drugs or increased dosages of current medications. Nutritional changes, physical activity, electroconvulsive therapy (ECT), transcranial magnetic stimulation (TMS), and psychotherapy are examples of nonpharmacologic techniques that can be beneficial adjuncts to medication therapy to improve symptoms of depression. This article reviews some of the most common nonpharmacologic methods of treating

Department of Neuropsychiatry, DENT Neurologic Institute, 3980 Sheridan Drive, Amherst, NY 14226, USA
E-mail address: nmiller@dentinstitute.com

Physician Assist Clin 6 (2021) 395–410
https://doi.org/10.1016/j.cpha.2021.02.004
2405-7991/21/© 2021 Elsevier Inc. All rights reserved.
physicianassistant.theclinics.com

depression, provides an overview of how they work, and describes their effects on neurochemistry and efficacy.

BACKGROUND

Depression is a common and serious medical illness that negatively affects how a person thinks, feels, and acts. Depression affects more than 18 million people annually in the United States. However, only 50% of those affected seek treatment.[3] Depression is one of the leading causes of disability and contributes to substance abuse, job loss, and suicide.[4] Depression is often a chronic disease with a high probability of reoccurrence. Studies have shown that individuals with major depressive disorder (MDD) experience, on average, 4 major depressive episodes (MDEs) in their lifetimes, with around 25% having 6 MDEs or more.[5] However, MDD is treatable with a combination of medications and nonpharmacologic methods. Medications tend to be the most common form of treatment of depression. Because of the likelihood of reoccurrence during a patient's lifetime, nonpharmacologic techniques can improve long-term success. Interventions such as cognitive behavior therapy (CBT) decrease the risk of relapse after remission of depressive symptoms.[6]

For a diagnosis of depression to be considered, 5 or more of the following symptoms must be present in the same 2-week period[7]:

- Feeling sad or having a depressed mood
- Markedly diminished interest or pleasure in all or almost all activities
- Appetite changes leading to weight loss or gain unrelated to dieting (>5% change in a month)
- Trouble sleeping or sleeping too much
- Loss of energy or increased fatigue
- Increase in purposeless physical activity (eg, hand-wringing or pacing) or slowed movements and speech (actions observable by others)
- Feeling worthless or guilty
- Difficulty thinking, concentrating, or making decisions
- Thoughts of death or suicide

Depressive symptoms may be mild to severe and may persist for several months or, in severe cases, years. To qualify as an MDD diagnosis, these symptoms must represent a change from previous functioning and at least 1 of the symptoms must be (1) depressed mood or (2) loss of interest or pleasure in activities. These symptoms must not be attributed to the use of a substance or another medical condition. Symptoms often cause significant distress or impairments in social, occupational, or other important areas of functioning. There can be several severe types of depression, including irrational, psychotic, or even delusional symptoms.[8] However, MDD cannot be diagnosed if the occurrence of the major depressive episode is better explained by a schizoaffective disorder, schizophrenia, schizophreniform disorder, delusional disorder, another specified disorder on the schizophrenia spectrum, or other psychotic disorder. Furthermore, depression should not be diagnosed if there has ever been a manic or hypomanic episode in the patient's medical history, which would indicate a possible bipolar diagnosis.[9]

NEUROTRANSMITTERS

Depression has negative effects on brain structure, which can impair cognitive functioning.[10] Depression cannot be discussed without mentioning the neurotransmitters that are usually implicated: serotonin, norepinephrine, and dopamine. A neurotransmitter is a chemical used by the nervous system to send messages between nerve cells.[11] When sending and receiving chemical signals, the cells rely on changes in the electrical current, depolarization (a rapid change in electrical charge), to communicate with other neurons.

A neurotransmitter must meet several criteria[12]:

- It is a substance that is stored in a presynaptic neuron
- It must be released by depolarization, which is associated with the influx of Ca++ ions
- The substance must bind to a specific receptor on the postsynaptic neuron

Different types of neurons can affect the way a message is transmitted. There are inhibitory neurons, usually glutamate, and excitatory neurons, such as GABA (γ-aminobutyric acid). These neurons can change the electrical charge of the brain by affecting the polarity of a cell membrane.[8]

Serotonin is a neurotransmitter synthesized from the amino acid tryptophan through a series of chemical reactions.[13] It is a monoamine that can alter the activity of excitatory and inhibitory neurons. Serotonin is primarily linked to mood regulation but involves many other functions in the body: sleep, sexual functioning, blood clotting, and healthy digestion. Most of the body's serotonin is produced in the gut.[12] Changes in serotonin levels, at both the presynaptic and postsynaptic junctions, have been seen in depressed patients.[14] All of the serotonin in the central nervous system (CNS) is synthesized in the raphe nuclei neurons found in the pons, medulla, and midbrain.[15]

Norepinephrine, also known as noradrenaline, is both a neurotransmitter and a hormone. It is involved in attention modulation, sleep-wake cycles, and mood regulation.[15] Like serotonin, norepinephrine works as a neurotransmitter, passing signals from one nerve cell to another. As a hormone, norepinephrine works alongside epinephrine (adrenaline) to give the body sudden energy in times of stress, thereby activating the fight-or-flight response.[16] Norepinephrine is primarily stored in the locus cerulus, near the fourth ventricle in the pons, whereas small amounts are stored in the adrenal glands on top of the kidneys.[15,16] Early theories of the pathogenesis of depression focused on a relative deficiency of norepinephrine, which was largely caused by the observed mechanism of action of drugs such as imipramine.[14] It was theorized that too little norepinephrine leads to depressive symptoms, but excesses could lead to mania.

Dopamine is a catecholamine neurotransmitter like norepinephrine. It is synthesized from the amino acid tyrosine in dopaminergic nerve terminals.[17] Dopamine plays a critical role in motivational arousal, responsiveness to conditioned incentive stimuli, and reward prediction.[18,19] It has nerve cells in the midbrain and axons that stretch to various other areas of the brain. Dopaminergic pathways allow dopamine to travel to different regions of the brain. There are 3 main pathways: mesostriatal, mesolimbic, and mesocortical. Alterations in these pathways can lead to delusions, hallucinations, aggressive behavior, motor function disturbances, and/or cognitive changes.[15,17]

INFLAMMATION AND DIET

An imbalance in neurotransmitters in the brain can lead to depression, but chronic emotional and physical stress can also contribute. Tension in the body leads to the sympathetic nervous system's activation, initiating a fight-or-flight response. In turn, this generates an inflammatory immune response in preparation to fight off any incoming threats.[20] Inflammation can lead to or even exacerbate depression.[21]

Many factors can cause inflammation. One is adiposity or obesity. Adipose tissue is a source of inflammatory factors, which include adipokines, chemokines, and cytokines.[22] Adipose tissues' primary role is to store triglycerides and release free fatty acids during fasting.[23] Obesity is an inflammatory condition in which adipocytes contribute to increased levels of proinflammatory cytokines.[23] Obesity is often caused by a sedentary lifestyle and the consumption of processed foods high in fats and sugars. Systemic inflammation leads to insulin resistance and type 2 diabetes. Chronic neuroinflammation by inflammatory cytokines, such as interleukin (IL)-6, IL-1, and tumor necrosis factor alpha, can lead to reduced metabolism of neurotransmitters. In turn, this leads to decreased serotonin, dopamine, and norepinephrine concentrations in the brain, resulting in increased depressive symptoms.[24] Exercise can be beneficial in improving systemic inflammation by reducing adipose tissue.[25] Regular physical activity is vital to healing disorders of both the body and the mind.

Proper nutrition is crucial in the treatment of depression. Diets should encompass a wide variety of fruits, vegetables, high-quality protein, and vitamins and minerals such as folate, B-complex vitamins, and omega-3 fatty acids.[26] A Mediterranean diet encompasses all of these nutrients; omega-3 fatty acids, specifically eicosapentaenoic acid and docosahexaenoic acid, as well as vitamin B_{12} and folate supplementation. These dietary additions to the daily diet have been shown to decrease the risk of depression.[27] In some cases, depression has been associated with reduced levels of neurotransmitters in the CNS, including serotonin, dopamine, norepinephrine, and GABA. If an individual's depressive symptoms seem to be caused by low serotonin levels, it may be hypothesized that these symptoms may be lessened by increasing serotonin levels. Diets rich in the amino acids tryptophan, tyrosine, phenylalanine, and methionine have been shown to be helpful in treating mood disorders because they contain the building blocks of these essential neurotransmitters (Fig. 1).[26]

Tryptophan is converted to serotonin in the body through a series of chemical reactions.[26] It has been suggested that a diet rich in tryptophan along with physical activity and other nonpharmacologic techniques might be beneficial in treating depression. Tryptophan-rich foods include beef, pork, cheese, soy products, squash seeds, and fish.[28] Studies to increase serotonin levels solely through a tryptophan-rich diet have not produced significant results and are inconclusive.[29]

Tyrosine is another critical amino acid in the treatment of depressive symptoms. It is converted to L-dopa (precursor of dopamine).[26] Through a series of chemical reactions, dopamine can be further converted into norepinephrine.[30] Dopamine and norepinephrine have been shown to boost motivational arousal and energy levels. Tyrosine can be found naturally in many foods, with the highest concentrations being found in poultry, fish, cheese, and beans. Tyrosine is also produced as phenylalanine, an essential amino acid, and is naturally converted to tyrosine in the liver and kidneys.[31]

Consuming a diet high in sugar or processed foods can also lead to inflammation. Metabolism of sugar consequently leads to the production of free fatty acids. Free fatty acids are stored in and released from adipose tissue.[32] The intake of high levels of dietary fats leads to inflammation because this promotes the translocation of gut microbes into the bloodstream.[33] The introduction of these endotoxins into the blood causes an inflammatory response which, in turn, intensifies symptoms of depression. Diets rich in foods with high glycemic index have been linked to increased inflammatory responses leading to an increased release of inflammatory cytokines and increased levels of free fatty acids.[34] The consumption of foods high in fats and sugars can also lead to insulin resistance and consequently increases the risk of developing

Amino Acids Essential for Neurotransmitter production

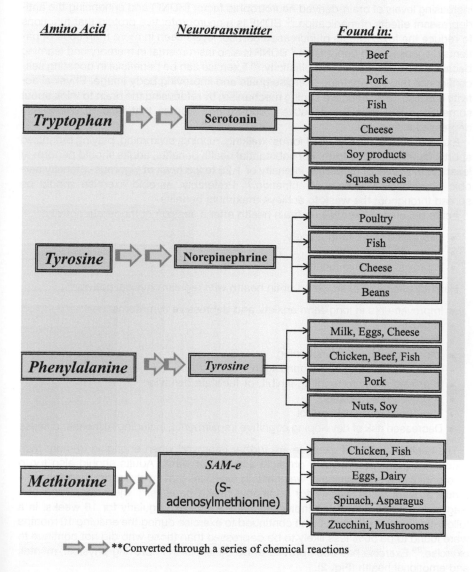

Amino Acid   *Neurotransmitter*   *Found in:*

Tryptophan ⇨⇨ **Serotonin** — Beef / Pork / Fish / Cheese / Soy products / Squash seeds

Tyrosine ⇨⇨ **Norepinephrine** — Poultry / Fish / Cheese / Beans

Phenylalanine ⇨⇨ **Tyrosine** — Milk, Eggs, Cheese / Chicken, Beef, Fish / Pork / Nuts, Soy

Methionine ⇨⇨ **SAM-e** (S-adenosylmethionine) — Chicken, Fish / Eggs, Dairy / Spinach, Asparagus / Zucchini, Mushrooms

⇨ ⇨ ****Converted through a series of chemical reactions**

Fig. 1. Amino acids essential for neurotransmitter production and the common foods in which they are found.

diabetes. The increased sugar levels in the blood may lead to increased fatigue and thus exacerbate feelings of depression.

PHYSICAL ACTIVITY

Physical activity can be defined as any activity that works the muscles and uses energy. It does not have to be running, organized sports, or overly strenuous. However, it should be consistent and performed regularly to achieve maximum benefits. Exercise can help alleviate depressive symptoms by improving neuroplasticity by increasing levels of brain-derived neurotrophic factor (BDNF) and enhancing the antidepressant effects of medication.[35] BDNF is a neuroprotective protein that functions to reduce the toxic effects of increased cortisol levels seen in more than 60% of patients diagnosed with depression.[3] BDNF is also instrumental in memory and learning because of its effects on neuroplasticity.[36] Exercise can be beneficial in boosting self-confidence through attaining exercise goals and improving body image. Physical activity can also be an effective coping mechanism by refocusing the brain to think about something other than the negative thoughts and worries that tend to overwhelm depressed individuals.

Exercise comes in a myriad of forms: walking, running, swimming, playing organized sports, dancing, and so forth. For substantial health benefits, adults should perform at least 2.5 to 5 h/wk of moderate-intensity or 1.25 to 2.5 h/wk of vigorous-intensity aerobic physical activity or a combination.[37] Preferably, aerobic exercise should be spread throughout the week to achieve maximum benefits.

Acute benefits of exercise on brain health after a session of moderate activity[37]:

- Decreased short-term anxiety
- Improved sleep
- Improved cognitive function

Habitual effects of exercise on brain health with regular physical activity[37]:

- Improvements in long-term anxiety and depressive symptoms
- Improved deep sleep
- Improved quality of life
- Improved executive functioning
- Improved planning and organization
- Improved ability to monitor, inhibit, or facilitate behaviors
- Improved task initiation
- Improved emotional control
- Decreased risk of developing cognitive impairments, including Alzheimer disease

The health benefits of exercise are further improved when engaging in more than 5 hours of moderate-intensity physical activity per week. Adults should also try to incorporate strength training or weightlifting exercises that involve more than 1 muscle group at least twice weekly for additional health benefits.[37] Blumenthal and colleagues[38] studied depressed individuals who exercised regularly for 16 weeks. In a follow-up study, participants who continued to exercise during the ensuing 10 months were found to be 50% less likely to be depressed than those who did not continue to exercise.[39] Exercise has been proved to be beneficial in improving physical, mental, and emotional health (Fig. 2).

Yoga is a specific exercise that can provide health benefits for both the body and the mind without being overly taxing to the body. It is a popular health practice with roots in Indian philosophy that combines elements of meditation, physical postures, and rhythmic breathing for a unique mind-body experience. Yoga has been shown to improve flexibility, decrease stress, increase BDNF levels in the brain/body, and decrease cortisol levels.[40] The modifiable nature of yoga lends itself to individuals with limited mobility and different clinical diagnoses and is suitable for all age groups. There have been positive correlations between yoga practice and improvements in diabetes, cardiovascular function, and various musculoskeletal conditions.[10] Yoga requires mental focus to simultaneously work through physical postures, meditation,

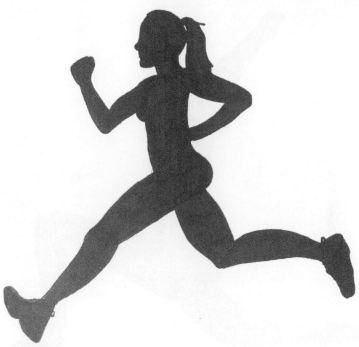

Fig. 2. For substantial health benefits, adults should perform at least 2.5 to 5 h/wk of moderate-intensity aerobic activity. Running is one such exercise to facilitate improvements in health and well-being.

and breathing exercises. As the mind becomes better able to focus, self-awareness tends to improve. This type of practice and mental focus may improve cognitive function, attention, and memory[10] (**Fig. 3**).

Imaging studies with MRI, functional MRI and single-photon emission computed tomography (SPECT) have shown improvements in brain structure and function in yoga practitioners. Several changes were noted in the brains of yoga practitioners[10]:

- Increased cortical thickening in the left prefrontal cortex
- Increased volume of the left hippocampus
- Increased size of several regions of the brain (frontal, limbic, temporal, occipital, cerebellar)
- Decreased activation of the dorsolateral prefrontal cortex during working memory

Yoga has also been shown to increase BDNF levels in the brain and decrease serum cortisol levels, thereby improving depression.[40]

BRAIN STIMULATION THERAPIES

Outside of exercise and nutrition, several brain stimulation techniques can be used as adjunctive therapies to help mitigate depressive symptoms. Two of the most common are electroconvulsive therapy (ECT) and TMS.

The earliest brain stimulation techniques involved live fish. The ancient Greeks and Romans used the shocking powers of Nile catfish and electric rays to treat headaches and various other medical ailments.[41] They placed live fish across the patient's brow

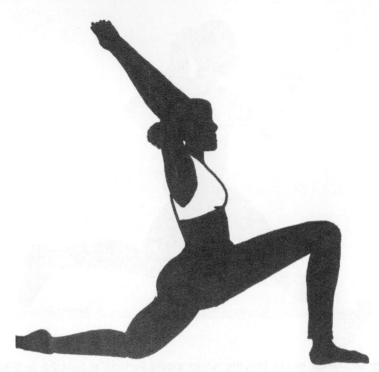

Fig. 3. Anjaneyasana (or crescent lunge) is a yoga pose that incorporates the muscles of the entire body, providing stretching, strengthening, balance, and stability. It is sometimes referred to as Salutation pose.

or had the patients stand on several fish at once, causing the fish to discharge their powers. It was not until many centuries later that these powers were discovered to be electricity. It would not be until the eighteenth century that machines were invented and marketed that could produce electricity on demand.[41]

In 1938, Italian physician Ugo Cerletti was the first clinician to use ECT as a treatment of a psychiatric patient. Dr Cerletti was able to develop a safer, improved mechanism for inducing seizures using electricity.[42] Before this, pharmacologically induced convulsive therapies, introduced in 1934, were common. However, these chemically induced seizures were painful, not easily controlled, and could lead to death or severe disability. Lobotomies, a type of neurosurgery that involved severing the connections within the brain, were also common during this time period. These procedures also came with inherent risks including incontinence, confusion, seizures, coma, and death.

ECT is highly effective in treating major depression. Evidence indicates that it can substantially improve symptoms in 80% of patients with uncomplicated severe depression.[43] The ECT procedure is administered by a team of medical professionals including an anesthesiologist, a psychiatrist, a nurse, and/or a physician assistant. Before the procedure, the patient is given a muscle relaxant and general anesthesia while electrodes are placed on the scalp. Electrical pulses stimulate the patient's brain, causing a short, controlled seizure that lasts approximately 1 minute. The patient is asleep while this occurs and wakes up after about 5 to 10 minutes[2] (**Fig. 4**). Patients typically receive ECT treatments 2 to 3 times per week up to 12 treatments, depending on the severity of symptoms. Patients are then managed with medications

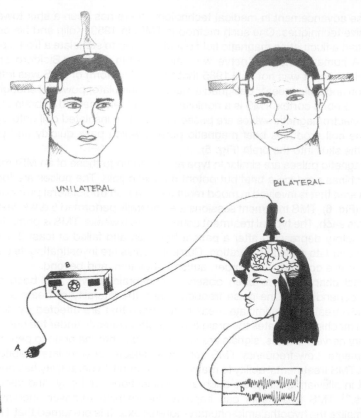

UNILATERAL

BILATERAL

Fig. 4. Unilateral and bilateral placement of electrodes for ECT, and ECT apparatus. Electrical current is obtained from power source in wall (A) and released through ECT machine (B). The current is then passed through electrodes on the scalp (C), inducing a seizure. An EEG (D) is commonly used from a nonparalyzed part of the body (eg, the foot) to document the seizure.

and/or psychotherapy. Some may need to return for maintenance ECT treatments. ECT is used not only in severe depression but also in patients experiencing mania, catatonia, or life-threatening conditions in need of emergent resolution.

ECT improves depressive symptoms by giving patients a mental reset of sorts. ECT reduces metabolism in the prefrontal and parietal regions of the brain. The reductions in metabolism correlate with treatment outcomes. Both bioelectric suppression immediately after seizure termination and the magnitude of delta activity in prefrontal regions in the interictal electroencephalogram (EEG), have been associated with superior ECT outcomes, suggesting that reductions in neural activity may be critical to efficacy.[44]

Some investigators have hypothesized that depression is caused by aberrant electrical activity within the brain, so the antidepressant effect of ECT may be caused by its ability to calm the mind's electrical activity. Depression may also be caused by a loss of BDNF, which results in a decrease in activity in the neural networks that regulate mood. Stimulation therapies such as ECT, TMS, and vagus nerve stimulation increase BDNF levels, thereby improving depressive symptoms.[41]

With the advancement in medical technology, there has been a shift toward more noninvasive techniques. One such method is TMS. In 1959, Kolin and his coworkers showed that a fluctuating magnetic field could be used to stimulate a frog's peripheral muscle. A human peripheral nerve was stimulated in 1965 by Bickford and Flemming.[45] However, it was not until 1985 that the modern form of TMS was introduced. O'Reardon and colleagues[46] designed a magnetic stimulator powerful enough to stimulate the cerebral cortex. TMS is a noninvasive treatment method of brain stimulation in which electromagnetic waves are passed through an insulated coil onto a patient's scalp. The coil produces brief magnetic pulses, which pass quickly and painlessly through the skull into the brain (**Fig. 5**).

The magnetic pulses are similar in type and strength to those of an MRI machine.[47] TMS machines produce a brief but potent magnetic field. The pulses are focused on the brain area that is involved in mood regulation, the left dorsolateral prefrontal cortex (DLPFC) (**Fig. 6**). TMS treatment sessions are generally performed 5 d/wk, lasting 20 to 40 minutes each. The typical treatment course is 5 to 6 weeks. TMS is primarily used to treat refractory depression after a patient has tried and failed at least 2 antidepressants at adequate dose and duration. Current studies are investigating its use in anxiety, obsessive compulsive disorder, autism, addiction, and beyond.

Neuronal changes have been observed and brain activity has been shown to improve depending on the pulse frequency and the laterality of treatment (right vs left).[48] TMS treatments stimulate areas of the brain that are affected by depression. The TMS machine stimulates the brain tissue (cortex) directly under the coils. Through secondary nerve impulses, signals are carried deeper into the brain to perform further improvements. Low-frequency TMS can more selectively stimulate inhibitory GABA neurons. TMS treatments' ability to manipulate neuronal hyperactivity has been shown to assist in alleviating disorders such as hallucinations, epilepsy, and various panic disorders.[41] TMS treatments can improve monoamine turnover, increase BDNF, and normalize the hypothalamic-pituitary-adrenal axis. It is presumed that TMS works

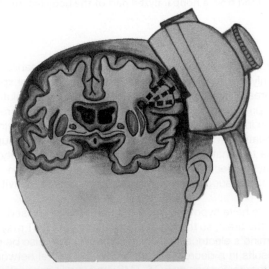

Fig. 5. TMS coil. Magnetic fields generated by the TMS coil induce a change in the brain's electrical current just below the skull.

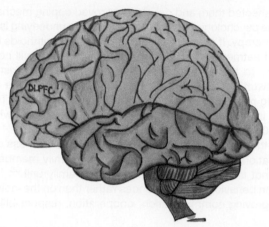

Fig. 6. DLPFC. TMS pulses are directed at this particular area of the brain because it is involved in mood regulation.

to alter the molecular environment of the CNS by activating various networks within the brain.[41]

Psychotherapy

Psychotherapy, or talk therapy, helps people with mental illness or emotional difficulties work through difficult issues or problems. Treatment goals are to eliminate or control symptoms to allow people to live happier, healthier, and more productive lives. Psychologists use scientifically validated procedures and therapies to help patients develop more robust, effective coping strategies.[49] This type of treatment only works if both the psychotherapist and the patient collaborate and talk openly without judgment. Psychotherapy is a modality grounded in dialogue and is meant to be supportive, objective, and neutral.[49]

CBT and interpersonal therapy (IPT), among other types of therapy, have been shown to alter brain function in clients with depression.[50] CBT is a form of therapy that focuses on recognizing negative thoughts and beliefs and works to correct them. Patients with depression may have feelings and thoughts that exacerbate their depressive symptoms by sustained distorted thought processing. Patients may dwell on the negative aspects of social interactions that perpetuate the symptoms of depression.[51] These thoughts are obstacles to their recovery, and CBT allows patients to recognize these thoughts as falsehoods and work toward changing their thought process. Counselors work with patients to revise thought patterns and develop a more realistic perception of themselves and the world around them, resulting in more positive interactions and relationships.[52] CBT has been shown to reduce the risk of relapse of depression by 14% to 22%.[6] Studies have shown that telephone sessions of CBT may reduce depressive symptoms further than regular in-person meetings because of convenience, patient comfort, and the ability to conduct the session at home.[24]

IPT is another form of psychotherapy in which the therapist works with the patient to identify key interpersonal relationships that may have caused depressive symptoms.[52] This therapy is most effective for depressed patients in whom a specific event (the death of a loved one, end of a relationship, or loss of a job) caused the depression. Therapists focus on 1 or 2 events and work with the patients to identify how these events negatively affected them and develop improved coping mechanisms. Psychotherapy requires the psychologist to identify the patient's underlying issue to select the most appropriate therapy. If a patient is not honest with or withholds information from the therapist, this treatment modality may be ineffective and will not produce long-term improvements to the patient's overall condition. Characteristics of empathy, genuineness, trustworthiness, and the ability to communicate are all cornerstones of effective, helping relationships between client and counselor.[52] Therapy sessions can be conducted in individual, couple, family, or group sessions, with sessions usually lasting 30 to 60 minutes weekly.[53]

Family systems therapy (FST) addresses the interconnectedness of an individual's problem to the relationship and interactions between family members.[54] An individual's choices are not isolated and contribute to the family unit.[55] The focus of this type of therapy is on behavioral consequences rather than on the individual. The goals of FST include improving communication, cooperation, responsibilities, and coping strategies.[55]

Person-centered therapy is an approach that allows clients to determine the direction of therapy and the goals they wish to achieve. It is based on the theory that individuals have the capacity for self-healing.[56] It theorizes that clients respond to stressors or events based on their environment. The goals of person-centered therapy are to promote self-awareness and responsibility, and empower clients to have confidence in themselves and their decisions.[57]

A Finnish study by Lehto and colleagues[58] took patients with MDD and randomized them to receive short-term psychodynamic psychotherapy or fluoxetine. A PET scan was obtained before and 4 months after treatment. The group that received psychotherapy showed an increase in 5-HT1A (5-hydroxytryptamine) receptor density, whereas the group that received medication showed no change. The patients also underwent SPECT and MRI scanning for comparison. There was an increase in serotonin transporters in patients with atypical depression that received psychotherapy.[58] It has been shown that there is no significant difference in efficacy between various types of psychotherapy. Psychotherapy and psychopharmacology have shown comparable rates of effectiveness. However, when these 2 modalities are combined, they are significantly more effective than pharmacotherapy alone.[52]

SUMMARY

Many modalities can be used as successful adjuncts to treat depressive symptoms in combination with medication. There are basic techniques, including improving nutritional intake or engaging in physical activity. Psychotherapy, ECT, and TMS are more advanced methods. All of these have been proved to decrease depressive symptoms alone or in combination with medication. To achieve the maximum benefits in the treatment of depression, it is essential to establish a trusting relationship with the patient to best determine the proper modality for each individual.

CLINIC CARE POINTS

- Pharmacotherapy should almost never be used as monotherapy
- Pharmacologic intervention in addition to pharmacotherapy is more beneficial in alleviating depressive symptoms than medication alone
- Exercise has been proved to decrease obesity, cortisol levels, and inflammation
- Inflammation can lead to increased depressive symptoms due to decreased quantity of neurotransmitters

- Yoga has been shown to increase brain structure and function as well as BDNF levels
- ECT is the gold standard treatment of refractory depression
- Properly balanced diets, such as the Mediterranean diet, are important for physical and mental health
- Tryptophan-rich diets have not been proved to improve depressive symptoms by increasing serotonin levels

ACKNOWLEDGMENTS

Megan Sackett illustrated the figures provided in this article.

DISCLOSURE

The author has nothing to disclose.

REFERENCES

1. Trindade E, Menon D, Topfer LA, et al. Adverse effects associated with selective serotonin reuptake inhibitors and tricyclic antidepressants: a meta-analysis. CMAJ 1998;159(10):1245–52.
2. Demyttenaere K, Enzlin P, Dewé W, et al. Compliance with antidepressants in a primary care setting, 1: beyond lack of efficacy and adverse events. J Clin Psychiatry 2001;62(Suppl 22):30–3.
3. Preston J, O'Neal JH, Talaga MC. Depressive disorders. In: Handbook of clinical psychopharmacology for therapists. Oakland (CA): New Harbinger Publications, Incorporated; 2017. p. 79–91.
4. Reichenberg LW, Seligman L. Depressive disorders. In: Selecting effective treatments: a comprehensive systematic guide to treating mental disorders. Hoboken (NJ): John Wiley & Sons, Inc; 2016. p. 146–66.
5. Angst J. The epidemiology of depressive disorders. Eur Neuropsychopharmacol 1995;5(Suppl):95–8.
6. Clarke K, Mayo-Wilson E, Kenny J, et al. Can non-pharmacological interventions prevent relapse in adults who have recovered from depression? A systematic review and meta-analysis of randomised controlled trials. Clin Psychol Rev 2015; 39:58–70.
7. Parekh R. What is depression?. 2017. Available at: https://www.psychiatry.org/patients-families/depression/what-is-depression. Accessed June 8, 2020.
8. Papolos DF. The personal experience. In: Overcoming depression. Site of publication not identified. New York: Harpercollins; 1998. p. 5–30.
9. American Psychiatric Association. Desk reference to the diagnostic criteria from DSM-5. Arlington (VA): American Psychiatric Association; 2013. p. 94–5.
10. Gothe NP, Khan I, Hayes J, et al. Yoga effects on brain health: a systematic review of the current literature. Brain Plast 2019;5(1):105–22.
11. Higgins ES, George MS. Cells and circuits. In: The neuroscience of clinical psychiatry: the pathophysiology of behavior and mental illness. Philadelphia: Wolters Kluwer; 2019. p. 28–39.
12. Higgins ES, George MS. Neurotransmitters. In: The neuroscience of clinical psychiatry: the pathophysiology of behavior and mental illness. Philadelphia: Wolters Kluwer; 2019. p. 41–7.

13. Charney DS, Nestler EJ, Deutch A. Neurochemical systems in the central nervous system. In: Charney DS, Nestler EJ, editors. Neurobiology of mental illness. Oxford (United Kingdom): Oxford University Press; 2004. p. 12–23.
14. Charney DS, Nestler EJ, Steven GJ, et al. The neurochemistry of depressive disorders: clinical studies. In: Charney DS, Nestler EJ, editors. Neurobiology of mental illness. Oxford (United Kingdom): Oxford University Press; 2004. p. 441–53.
15. Blumenfeld H. Brainstem III: internal structures and vascular supply. In: Neuroanatomy through clinical cases. New York: Sinauer Associates/Oxford University Press; 2021. p. 630–7.
16. Rogers K. Norepinephrine. Encyclopædia Britannica. 2020. Available at: https://www.britannica.com/science/norepinephrine. Accessed July 16, 2020.
17. Stahl SM. Psychosis and schizophrenia. In: Stahl's essential psychopharmacology: neuroscientific basis and practical applications. Cambridge (United Kingdom): Cambridge University Press; 2013. p. 86–96.
18. Salamone JD, Correa M, Mingote S, et al. Nucleus accumbens dopamine and the regulation of effort in food-seeking behavior: implications for studies of natural motivation, psychiatry, and drug abuse. J Pharmacol Exp Ther 2003;305(1):1–8.
19. Schultz W. Predictive reward signal of dopamine neurons. J Neurophysiol 1998; 80(1):1–27.
20. Won E, Kim YK. Stress, the autonomic nervous system, and the immune-kynurenine pathway in the etiology of depression. Curr Neuropharmacol 2016; 14(7):665–73.
21. Higgins ES, George MS. Immunity and inflammation. In: The neuroscience of clinical psychiatry: the pathophysiology of behavior and mental illness. Philadelphia: Wolters Kluwer; 2019. p. 113–6.
22. Shelton RC, Miller AH. Inflammation in depression: is adiposity a cause? Dialogues Clin Neurosci 2011;13(1):41–53.
23. Makki K, Froguel P, Wolowczuk I. Adipose tissue in obesity-related inflammation and insulin resistance: cells, cytokines, and chemokines. ISRN Inflamm 2013; 2013:139239.
24. Liu Q, Li R, Qu W, et al. Pharmacological and non-pharmacological interventions of depression after traumatic brain injury: a systematic review. Eur J Pharmacol 2019;865:172775.
25. Woods JA, Wilund KR, Martin SA, et al. Exercise, inflammation and aging. Aging and disease. 2012. Available at: https://www.ncbi.nlm.nih.gov/pmc/articles/PMC3320801. Accessed May 15, 2020.
26. Rao TS, Asha MR, Ramesh BN, et al. Understanding nutrition, depression and mental illnesses. Indian J Psychiatry 2008;50(2):77–82.
27. Popa TA, Ladea M. Nutrition and depression at the forefront of progress. J Med Life 2012;5(4):414–9.
28. Strasser B, Gostner JM, Fuchs D. Mood, food, and cognition: role of tryptophan and serotonin. Curr Opin Clin Nutr Metab Care 2016;19(1):55–61.
29. Richard DM, Dawes MA, Mathias CW, et al. Basic metabolic functions, behavioral research and therapeutic indications. Int J Tryptophan Res 2009;2:45–60.
30. Molinoff PB, Axelrod J. Biochemistry of catecholamines. Annu Rev Biochem 1971;40:465–500.
31. Kohlmeier M. Amino acids and nitrogen compounds. In: Handbook of nutrient metabolism. Oxford (England): Academic; 2003. p. 214–321.
32. Boden G. Obesity and free fatty acids. Endocrinol Metab Clin North Am 2008; 37(3):635–ix.

33. Fritsche KL. The science of fatty acids and inflammation. Adv Nutr 2015;6(3): 293S–301S.
34. Della Corte KW, Perrar I, Penczynski KJ, et al. Effect of dietary sugar intake on biomarkers of subclinical inflammation: a systematic review and meta-analysis of intervention studies. Nutrients 2018;10(5):606.
35. Mura G, Moro MF, Patten SB, et al. Exercise as an add-on strategy for the treatment of major depressive disorder: a systematic review. CNS Spectr 2014;19(6): 496–508.
36. BDNF gene - Genetics Home Reference - NIH. U.S. National Library of Medicine. 2013. Available at: https://ghr.nlm.nih.gov/gene/BDNF. Accessed June 24, 2020.
37. Physical Activity Basics. Centers for Disease Control and Prevention. 2020. Available at: https://www.cdc.gov/physicalactivity/basics/index.htm?CDC_AA_refVal=https%3A%2F%2Fwww.cdc.gov%2Fphysicalactivity%2Feveryone%2Fguidelines%2Findex.html. Accessed June 1, 2020.
38. Blumenthal JA, Babyak MA, Moore KA, et al. Effects of exercise training on older patients with major depression. Arch Intern Med 1999;159(19):2349–56.
39. Babyak M, Blumenthal JA, Herman S, et al. Exercise treatment for major depression: maintenance of therapeutic benefit at 10 months. Psychosom Med 2000; 62(5):633–8.
40. Naveen GH, Varambally S, Thirthalli J, et al. Serum cortisol and BDNF in patients with major depression-effect of yoga. Int Rev Psychiatry 2016;28(3):273–8.
41. Higgins ES, George MS. Brain stimulation therapies for clinicians. Washington, DC: American Psychiatric Pub.; 2009. p. 3, 30-40, 49-51, 60-62, 99-110.
42. Aruta A. Shocking waves at the museum: the Bini-Cerletti electro-shock apparatus. Med Hist 2011;55(3):407–12.
43. McDonald W. What is Electroconvulsive therapy (ECT)? What is ECT?. 2019. Available at: https://www.psychiatry.org/patients-families/ect. Accessed June 15, 2020.
44. Nobler MS, Oquendo MA, Kegeles LS, et al. Decreased regional brain metabolism after ect. Am J Psychiatry 2001;158(2):305–8.
45. Ilmoniemi RJ, Ruohonen J, Karhu J. Transcranial magnetic stimulation–a new tool for functional imaging of the brain. Crit Rev Biomed Eng 1999;27(3–5):241–84.
46. O'Reardon JP, Altinay M, Cristancho P. A new treatment option for major depression. Psychiatric Times 2010. Available at: https://www.psychiatrictimes.com/view/new-treatment-option-major-depression. Accessed June 29, 2020.
47. ECT and TMS in the Brain Stimulation Program at Johns Hopkins Hospital in Baltimore, Maryland. 2020. Available at: https://www.hopkinsmedicine.org/psychiatry/specialty_areas/brain_stimulation. Accessed June 16, 2020.
48. McClintock SM, Reti IM, Carpenter LL, et al. Consensus recommendations for the clinical application of repetitive Transcranial Magnetic Stimulation (rTMS) in the treatment of depression. J Clin Psychiatry 2018;79(1):16cs10905.
49. What is Psychotherapy? American Psychological Association. 2020. Available at: https://www.apa.org/helpcenter/understanding-psychotherapy. Accessed June 23, 2020.
50. Karlson H. How psychotherapy changes the brain. Psychiatric Times 2011. Available at: https://www.psychiatrictimes.com/view/how-psychotherapy-changes-brain. Accessed June 1, 2020.
51. Scott J. Cognitive therapy for depression. Br Med Bull 2001;57:101–13.
52. Zubernis L, Snyder M. Depressive disorders. In: Graves K, editor. Case conceptualization and effective interventions: assessing and treating mental, emotional, and behavioral disorders. Los Angeles (CA): Sage; 2016. p. 65–80.

53. Parekh R, Givon L. What is psychotherapy?. Available at: https://www.psychiatry. org/patients-families/psychotherapy. Accessed June 12, 2020.
54. Corey G. Family systems therapy. In: Theory and practice of counseling and psychotherapy. Boston: Cengage; 2017. p. 404–7.
55. Seligman L, Reichenberg LW. Family systems approaches. In: Theories of counseling and psychotherapy. India: Pearson; 2017. p. 390–401.
56. Corey G. Person centered therapy. In: Theory and practice of counseling and psychotherapy. Boston: Cengage; 2017. p. 165–7.
57. Seligman L, Reichenberg LW. Carl rogers and person-centered counseling. In: Theories of counseling and psychotherapy. Tamil Nadu: Pearson; 2017. p. 144–65.
58. Lehto SM, Tolmunen T, Joensuu M, et al. Changes in midbrain serotonin transporter availability in atypically depressed subjects after one year of psychotherapy. Prog Neuropsychopharmacol Biol Psychiatry 2008;32(1):229–37.

Mental Health and the Law

Brenda S. Fisher, PA-C, JD[a], Kerrigan LeBoeuf, BSN, RN[b],*

KEYWORDS

• Insanity plea • Sleepwalking • Legal defense

KEY POINTS

• The origin and revisions of the insanity plea.
• Review of some types of insanity pleas used in court.
• How courts interpret the insanity defense.

INTRODUCTION

Mental illness and the law governing the criminal who invokes *"mental illness"* as the cause is a complex subject. The jurors, prosecutors, defense attorneys, courts, and psychiatry all try to determine when a person is so mentally disturbed he/she should not be held accountable for their acts. The courts must decide if the defendant is competent to stand trial. A comprehensive review of all the interactions with law and mental health would take multiple books. Details of the laws, changes, and growth over time along with state-to-state variation can be overwhelming. I have chosen to look at the insanity plea, differences in the legal types of insanity definitions, and state-specific issues, highlighting how the courts and psychiatry have handled them.

COMPETENCY VERSUS CAPACITY

Within our practices we have to make decisions about a patient's ability to make decisions or to care for himself. This is not to say we judge competency. Competency is a legal term that encompasses all the person's affairs. The clinician decides capacity to decide and the courts decide competency. The beginning of all trials with an insanity claim starts with a decision of *"is the defendant competent to stand trial."*

Competency and capacity are similar terms but have different definitions. Competency is a global decision of impairment dealing with finances, wills, and trials. Competency is a legal term. To be competent to stand trial the defendant must be capable

---

[a] Medical Staff Advent Health Gordon, Virginia Bar Association, Hospitalist Office, 1035 Red Bud Rd NE, Calhoun, GA 30701, USA; [b] Floyd Home Care, Member of LHC Group, 101 E 2nd Ave, Suite 200, Rome, GA 30161, USA
* Corresponding author.
E-mail address: kmleboeuf@gmail.com

Physician Assist Clin 6 (2021) 411–419
https://doi.org/10.1016/j.cpha.2021.03.004
2405-7991/21/© 2021 Elsevier Inc. All rights reserved.
physicianassistant.theclinics.com

of understanding the nature and purpose of the proceedings taken against them. They must be able to assist their attorney with their defense.[1]

Capacity is cognition and is a medical decision. Determining capacity has 4 elements:

1. Be able to demonstrate understanding of the benefits and risks
2. Demonstrate appreciation of benefits and risks as well as alternatives
3. Show reasoning in making a decision
4. Communicate their choice to others

The medical community evaluates these elements and decides if the patient has capacity to make a medical decision.[2] In making this determination, barriers (ie, hearing or vision impairment) must be evaluated and reversed as appropriate. Any medical encephalopathy or drug intoxication that can be reversed must be done so before a determination of capacity.[2]

In deciding criminal liability, courts have to decide if the person is competent to stand trial. As noted earlier, they also decide if the defendant has the ability to understand the purpose of the proceedings and if he/she is able to assist the defense attorney.

In the case of *Mark Berberian and Emanuel Berberian v Diana Lynn*, the defendant suffered from dementia.[3] The question was could a patient with dementia be found responsible for harming his caregiver at the home where he was institutionalized. His past medical history showed advanced dementia with known tendencies of violent outbursts when agitated. The court noted that a patient with Alzheimer disease owed no duty to the nursing assistant to refrain from violent behavior because he did not have the capacity to control his behavior. The defendant could not be found guilty if the defense had proved to the jury that the defendant had such a diminished capacity that he could not appreciate the danger of his actions.[3] Note that the defense had the burden of proof for diminished capacity.

Harder to comprehend is the insanity plea by defendants. Courts have gone through evolutions in defining the insanity plea. For example, how can John Hinckley (attempted assignation of President Reagan to get Jodi Foster's attention) be found not guilty by reason of insanity and Jeffery Dahmer who stalked, killed, dismembered, and then ate them not be insane.[1] The question of responsibility for actions due to mental incompetence goes back to ancient religious traditions. Historians noted that demons became the cause of problems. It was believed by ancients that epilepsy was caused by demons. Around the tenth century it became *"the devil's sickness."* In early Roman law madness was punishment and so societal punishment was more lenient.[1]

DEVELOPMENT OF THE "MODERN" INSANITY DEFINITION

In the 1800s, England's Daniel M'Naghten felt persecuted by the Tories and set out to kill Sir Robert Peel, the Prime Minister. By accident he shot Edward Drummond, first to exit the Prime Minister's carriage. M'Naghten's defense was based on an insanity plea with moral perceptions being impaired.[1] Although he was acquitted, he spent 22 years in an insane asylum. English outrage over the verdict led to the *M'Naghten rule*. The basis of the rule is every man is presumed sane. To establish a defense of insanity, one must prove a defendant was laboring under a defect of reason regarding the committing act *at the time the act was committed*. If the defendant knew the nature of the act but he did not know it was wrong, he was able to use the insanity defense. In short *"a defect in reason caused by disease of the mind (mental illness), which impairs a person's ability to know the wrongfulness of one's conduct.*[4]*"*

With the United States, some states adopted this rule, whereas others thought it too narrow, New Hampshire being a prime example. In New Hampshire, *"An accused is not criminally responsible if his unlawful act was the product of mental disease or defect.[1]"* The goal was to use expert psychiatric testimony to help define the mental disease or defect.

Next, added to the definition of insanity was the *"Irresistible Impulse Test."* This focused on whether the mental illness or disease prevented the defendant from controlling his actions. In 1955, the American Law institute formulated the Model Penal Code. This was a combination of the M'Naghten rule and the irresistible impulse test stating:

> *A person is not responsible for criminal conduct if at the time of such conduct as a result of mental disease or defect he lacks substantial capacity either to appreciate the criminality [wrongfulness]of his conduct or to conform his conduct to the requirements of law.[4]*

After the Hinckley Jr's attempt on the President's life, Congress along with multiple states wanted to tighten up the insanity defense. In 1984, the *Insanity Defense Reform Act* was passed.[4] The Act contains 4 areas limiting the scope of insanity acquittals:

1. Under the new federal insanity test a defendant is not responsible for criminal conduct if, *"as a result of a severe mental disease or defect, [he] was unable to appreciate the nature and quality or the criminality or wrongfulness of his acts."* The act provides for a special verdict of *"not guilty only by reason of insanity."*
2. The burden of proof is shifted from the prosecutor to the defense who has the burden to prove the defendant's insanity by clear and convincing evidence. This is known as an affirmative defense in court.
3. Commitment of the acquitted defendant to the custody of the US Attorney General for treatment of a provisional term set at the maximum term of confinement authorized for the offense. The court does have option to revise the sentence if the defendant recovers mental capacity.
4. A new rule was introduced that barred specific testimony by expert witnesses directed to the mental state of a defendant at the time of the alleged act. The witness cannot give an opinion or inference as to whether the defendant did or did not have the mental state or condition constituting and element of the crime charged.

The rules were adopted by most states each with their own variations. The expert witness, the psychiatrist, has responsibility for fully evaluating the defendant and formulating opinions. As noted earlier, the expert cannot testify regarding the state of mind at the time of the act. Most of the insanity defenses require the defendant suffer from some form of psychological disorder or intellectual disability (previously referred to as mental retardation).

POSTTRAUMATIC STRESS DISORDER AND THE LAW

Some psychological disorders are harder to prove and are rarely used in court. One of these is posttraumatic stress disorder (PTSD). PTSD was first recognized after the Vietnam war although the disorder has been around for years under different names. In 1974, Patricia Hearst, then a 22-year-old newspaper heiress was kidnapped and participated in bank robbery. When she was released, her legal defense team used the term *"traumatic neurosis."* They tied this to her kidnapping by a terrorist group. More recently, PTSD is related to our war veterans. PTSD can be caused by stressful events that cause fear, loss of physical integrity, concern for death serious injury, and helplessness.[1]

Symptoms of PTSD can include flashbacks, nightmares, panic, and depression. In 2009, an Iraqi war veteran was found not guilty by reason of insanity due to PTSD by an Oregon trial court. The defendant presented evidence of a dissociative flashback causing him to kill an unarmed man. A dissociative flashback caused the defendant to lack the ability to conform his conduct to requirement of law during the attack. Proving mental state at the time of the incident can be very difficult for defendants.[1] To make it more complicated, every state has its own definition and limitations of the insanity defense.[4] In *Virger v The State and Cave v the State*, the Georgia court noted[5]:

> PTSD-like "explosive rage and fear which led to his unprovoked killing of an un-armed man" was properly excluded as irrelevant to the defendant's justification defense; relying on Thompson to affirm the exclusion of Dr. Loring's expert testimony that the defendant "could not form the requisite intent to commit the crimes charged because she suffered from PTSD".

> As we recognized in Thompson, Georgia takes a more restrictive position on this issue than many other jurisdictions, where the admission of evidence relating to a defendant's deficient mental condition to support defenses other than those based on diminished mental capacity or to negate a required element of a crime has been authorized by statute or judicial decision in at least some circumstances.

> We are not alone, however, in our adherence to the traditional position on this issue. For example, in State v. Mott, 187 Ariz. 536, 931 P.2d 1046 (1997), the defendant was charged with murder and child abuse based in part on not taking her daughter to a hospital after her boyfriend beat the child, who later died. The court also held that this limitation did not violate due process under the United States Constitution. We note that the United States Supreme Court has since held that Arizona's Mott rule does not violate due process "in restricting consideration of defense evidence of mental illness and incapacity to its bearing on a claim of insanity."

> If Georgia's longstanding law is to be changed to allow the admission of expert testimony in criminal cases to negate intent or otherwise support a mental capacity defense other than the ones now authorized by statute, that change should come from the General Assembly.[5]

Multiple Personality Defense

Another legal defense revolves around multiple personality disorder. The defendant claims it is the "other personality" who took control and thus the defendant has no memory of the event nor control over it. However, in *State v Grimsley* the court disagreed with the defense[6]:

> Assuming arguendo that the evidence was sufficient to establish such a complete break between appellant's consciousness as Robin and her consciousness as Jennifer that Jennifer alone was in control (despite years of therapy), nevertheless the evidence fails to establish the fact that Jennifer was either unconscious or acting involuntarily. There was only one person driving the car and only one person accused of drunken driving. It is immaterial whether she was in one state of consciousness or another, so long as in the personality then controlling her behavior, she was conscious and her actions were a product of her own volition. The evidence failed to demonstrate that Jennifer was unconscious or otherwise acting involuntarily.

Another branch of appellant's argument is that since Robin has only minimal recollection of what Jennifer did and was unable to respond to questions on the stand about the conduct constituting the offense, Robin was not conscious of that conduct and should not be held responsible for it. We are not persuaded. If we were to allow the bare existence of a defendant's multiple personality disorder to excuse criminal behavior, we would also relieve from responsibility for their criminal acts all defendants whose memories are blocked.[6]

The Hawaii Supreme Court, in *State v Rodriquez*, held each personality may or may not be criminally liable and each had to be examined under the state's test for insanity.[7] A different view was taken by the federal appeals court in *United States v Denny-Shaffer*. The defendant was convicted for kidnapping but appealed arguing she should be not guilty by reason of insanity because her dominant personality was not in control. The court held that multiple personality disorder qualified under the federal insanity definition. The court required that the defendant would have to prove the following at the time of the crime:

1. She was suffering from multiple personality disorder.
2. Her dominant personality was not in control and she was not aware that the alter personality was committing the offense.
3. Multiple personality disorder made the dominant personality unable to appreciate the nature and quality or wrongfulness of the conduct.

FUGUE, SOMNAMBULISM, AND SLEEPWALKING

Each state and the federal government can differ on the use of the insanity defense and the evidence required to the defense of insanity. The courts have looked at automatism, a state when the mind has no control over the actions of the body. This can happen in somnambulism, hypnosis, metabolic disorders, or fugue states. How courts handle these cases vary.

In 1878, a 28-year-old man with a long history of sleep terrors was tried for murder in Canada when he smashed his 18-month-old son against a wall one night. The defendant had been under stress and did not remember the act. He thought he was defending his family fighting off a wild beast. He was acquitted because he was unconscious of the nature of his act due to somnambulism.[8]

The idea that someone can perform complex tasks while sleepwalking is a difficult concept. In Arizona a man who had been under stress at work and having trouble sleeping was arrested for murder. He had come home from work and had dinner with his family. His family said there was an issue with the pool so he had looked at the pool. He put his tools in the trunk of his car because it had gotten dark and then went to bed. The next thing he remembers was the police at his door. They found his wife with multiple stab wounds and bloody knife and work clothes in his car. The next-door neighbor, on hearing screams and dogs barking, had looked out his window and saw the defendant putting on gloves and rolling a body into the pool; he immediately called the police. The defense stated the defendant was sleepwalking. Although he had a history of sleepwalking, he was convicted and sent to prison.[9] A sleepwalking defense is difficult in US courts.

A historical medical and legal review showed episodes of violent behavior that occurred with arousal from sleep were usually were directed at those in close proximity or who were encountered at the time of arousal.[10] Courts define sleepwalking as a state of unconsciousness or semiconscious so that the defendant is not performing a voluntary act. Thus, in Georgia, "*the Model Penal Code provides that a person who commits an act during unconsciousness or sleep has not committed a voluntary act and is not criminally responsible for the act. Moreover, LaFave notes that sleep-walking qualifies as such a defense."*[11]

A sleepwalking defense is not always easy to prove. Some juries find complex actions too detailed to attribute to sleepwalking. There is ongoing research to define the causes and to help understand the sleepwalking individual and his violent behavior (sleep walking violence).[9] Many similarities are noted in sleepwalking violence:

1. They occur soon after sleep arousal
2. The defendant has no history of violent behavior
3. The defendant has no memory of the event
4. The defendant has been under stress and has a history of sleep disturbances

If one looks at the unconscious defense, we have to look at other causes of unconsciousness such as drug and alcohol. Many defendants who note sleepwalking are also taking sleep medication, which can contribute to the sleep arousal and sleep walking. Are they then immune from guilt? As you can guess, courts can take different views.

In *Riley v Commonwealth of Virginia*, Riley had taken 3 or 4 sleeping pills, as well as an antihistamine and pain medications. He was involved in an accident resulting in bodily harm to the victim. After the accident, both the witnesses and the police officer noted he was incoherent and he failed a field sobriety test. His explanation to the officer was conflicting and confused. At the hospital, blood work showed no alcohol but evidence of diphenhydramine (Benadryl), propoxyphene (Darvon), and zolpidem (Ambien). When his fiancée returned home, she found the burners on the stove were on and food, his wallet, and phone were on the counter, but there was no sign of Riley. She reported that Riley had a history of a sleep disorder, seizures, and sleepwalking, although previously he had never left the apartment. Although Riley had been prescribed zaleplon (Sonata), he also had blister packs of zolpidem (Ambien) and eszopiclone (Lunesta) without proof of a prescription. A doctor testified at his trial that the blood level of zolpidem was too high for a single dose, but the antihistamine and pain medication level was as expected with a single dose. The physician also stated that Riley's behavior at the time of the accident could be caused by the high dose of zolpidem in combination with the other medications. The physician also stated sleep driving is a very rare occurrence although zolpidem has been noted to trigger sleep walking. The court found that the defendant voluntarily took an overdose of medication, knowing there were side effects. This voluntary use of nonprescribed drugs was an indiscriminate act that had the consequence of the accident, thus he was found guilty of voluntary intoxication.[12]

INTOXICATION

In *United States of America V Felix Garcia*, the court addressed voluntary intoxication. The defendant had known history of drug, alcohol abuse, and a diagnosis of bipolar disorder. After he started a fight brandishing a gun, police were called. As the police arrived, the defendant was riding bike away. Police pulled beside him to inquire about the incident. When Garcia pulled a gun on the officer, the officer fired striking Garcia in the stomach. During trial, Garcia was found competent via a psychiatric evaluation. Garcia pleaded insanity due to drug and alcohol use before the incident. The defense stated that the combination of bipolar disorder with drugs and alcohol had made Garcia unable to know or appreciate the quality of his actions. The court disagreed and noted that the voluntary ingestion of drugs and alcohol, even if they impaired his judgment of right and wrong, does not constitute an affirmative defense. A drug addict or alcoholic cannot use his addicted status as a defense.[13] The court stated that if substance abuse caused insanity, that would be a valid defense. However, there was no testimony showing defendants bipolar disorder was caused by his substance abuse and bipolar disorder does not meet criteria for severe mental illness.[13]

The court differentiates between chronic alcoholism and involuntary intoxication. The state of alcoholism is self-induced and the consumption is voluntary.[14] For involuntary intoxication, when you are given an unknown intoxicant or a practitioner prescribes a medication that unknowingly causes intoxication, you can claim the unconsciousness defense. However, in *Johnson v. Commonwealth*, the court made clear the limitations and effect of voluntary and involuntary intoxication.[15] Johnson had used corn whiskey for pain from a tooth while waiting to see a dentist. He stated he was involuntarily drunk and could not appreciate the wrongfulness of his actions. The court noted:

The law has always jealously guarded the effect of drunkenness as a defense in criminal cases, and even with all the restrictions surrounding it, the doctrine is a dangerous one and liable to be abused. We are not willing to render it more so by holding that an accused person can bring himself within the exception applicable in cases of involuntary intoxication by simply claiming that he drank intoxicants because he was suffering from pain or illness. ...such a precedent would open wide the door for false and fraudulent evasion of the general rule, and would in large measure destroy its efficiency. The rule has for ages been regarded as necessary for the safety of society, and its preservation and enforcement was never more important than under present conditions.

When people undertake, as the defendant in this case did, to prescribe for themselves and to select their own supply, they must be held responsible for the consequences. The only safe test of involuntary drunkenness, and the one almost if not quite universally found in the authorities, is the absence of an exercise of independent judgment and volition on the part of the accused in taking the intoxicant—as, for example, when he has been made drunk by fraudulent contrivance of others, by casualty, or by error of his physician.[15]

The Circuit Court of Virginia noted that the *Involuntary Intoxication* defense is a separate defense from the insanity plea. One has to prove that the intoxication was severe enough to make one unable to control their conduct and that one was unwillingly or unknowingly intoxicated.[16]

MENTAL ILLNESS

Courts in each state have variations on laws governing mental illness. Mental illness is recognized as a defense and must be proved by the defendant. The burden of proof can be "*clear and convincing evidence*" (a lower burden) or "*beyond a reasonable doubt*" depending on the state. In *Leland v State of Oregon*, the issue was burden of proof. In Oregon, the burden was "*beyond a reasonable doubt*," and the court ruled this higher level of proof did not violate the due process clause of the constitution.[17]

When a defendant is found criminally insane they can be confined to an institution for a period of time they would be incarcerated for their crime. However, if the institution finds a patient no longer needs psychiatric commitment and the time period of the crime is not served, is the defendant released to home of to prison? In *Commonwealth of Pennsylvania v Barnes*, the Supreme Court of Pennsylvania ruled on this issue. The defendant was guilty of involuntary manslaughter, sentenced to 6 years but was committed to the Philadelphia State Hospital. After 1 year, the Philadelphia State

Hospital thought the defendant was fit for discharge from the hospital. The defendant claimed she no longer had to serve the rest of her sentence. The court found that release from mental health treatment did not constitute entire satisfaction of the sentence. They moved her to prison with credit toward her sentence for time served in the mental institution.[18]

The scope of mental illness and the law is wide and far ranging. There are multiple intersections with mental disease and criminal behavior in this population. The main focus of the law is the ability to understand that the act was wrong, the consequences of the act, and/or the defendants' control over actions. Jurors have difficulty in finding not guilty due to insanity. The prosecution has to prove the essential elements of the crime beyond a reasonable doubt. Then the defendant has the burden of proof regarding insanity at the time of the commission of the crime.

The American Academy of Psychiatry and Law has practice guidelines for evaluation of defendants and testimony in court for defendants regarding the forensic examination. The American Psychiatric Association (APA) has objections to psychiatrists testifying regarding future mental health of a defendant. In the 1970s a psychiatrist by the name of Grigson testified frequently for the prosecution. He would testify in the penalty phase and give his opinion on the likelihood that the defendant would continue a life of crime. Grigson was famous for the number of defendants he sent to death row. However, one death row case was appealed to the US Supreme Court. In an amicus brief, the APA argued that psychiatrists should not testify in the penalty phase. The APA showed data that a psychiatrist has no expertise in predicting the future behavior of the defendant.[19] Since that case, psychiatrists do not testify in the penalty phase.

SUMMARY

Each state has its own laws governing the use of insanity, intoxication, and unconsciousness defenses. The laws and the medical knowledge are constantly changing as is all aspects of medicine; this makes it a difficult hurdle for the defense. Defendants face skepticism from the jurors and the court. Despite the skepticism, the obvious conclusion must be that the defendant was so affected by his mental state that he did not know right from wrong or that what he was doing was wrong for an insanity plea.

Many questions remain. How can the law and medical fields help those with mental illness before trouble? Can an inmate be forced to take medication for mental health? Mental health treatment is not always readily available, and those who need it may have physical, social, or mental roadblocks to obtaining help. Even if we do not think the law affects our everyday practice, it is both interesting and relevant. Understanding mental illness and legal issues as we treat patients in our practice is important. Even our most well-controlled patients can have an intersection with the legal community and we can hope for the best. And prepare for the worse.

CLINICS CARE POINTS

- Capacity is the medical definition and should be defined by the practitioner, while competency is a legal decision.
- It is important for a practiioner to identify psychiatric disease so the patient can get treatment.
- For practioners to recognize when they give out certain hypnotic medications, such as Ambien, it can have critical legal ramifications for their patients.

DISCLOSURE

None.

REFERENCES

1. Slovenko R. Psychiatry and criminal liability. Hoboken, (NJ): John Wiley and Sons, inc; 1995.
2. Barstow C, Shahan B, Roberts M. Evaluating medical decision-making capacity in practice. Am Fam Physician 2018;98(1):40–6.
3. Mark Berberian and Emanuel Berberian v Diana Lynn, AS guardian of Imcompetent Edmond Gerant in Superior Court of New Jersey, Appellate Division, 809A.2d 865; 355 N.J. Super. 210.
4. American Academy of Psychiatry and the Law (AAPL). AAPL Practice Guideline for forensic psychiatric evaluation of defendants raising the insanity defense. J Am Acad Psychiatry Law 2014;42(4 Suppl):S3–76.
5. Virger v The State, Cave v the State,824 S. E.2d 346, State v. Grimsley, 3 Ohio App.3d 265, 444 N.E.2d 1071, 3 OBR 308 (Ohio App. 1982)" 679 P2d 615, 67 Haw 70; Supreme Court of Hawaii, No.8865 March 8, 1984.
6. U.S. v Denny-Shaffer, 2 F3d999; 62 USLW 2167, No. 922144 U.S. Circuit Court of Appeals 10th Circuit.
7. Cartwright R. Sleepwalking violence: a sleep disorder, a legal dilemma, and a psychological challenge. Am J Psychiatry 2004;161(7):1149–58.
8. Pressman MR. Disorders of arousal from sleep and violent behavior: the role of physical contact and proximity. Sleep 2007;30(8):1039–47.
9. Smith v. State, 284 Ga. 33, 663 S.E.2d 155 (Ga. 2008) Brian Patrick Riley v Commonwealth of VA, Record No. 080920, Supreme Court of Appeals of Virginia, April 17, 2009.
10. United States of America v Felix Garcia 94 F3d 57 328NW 2d 836. 329 N.W.2d 833 (1983) State of Minnesota v James Michael Patch No. C7-81-1043 Supreme Court of Minnesota February 18, 1983.
11. Johnson v. Commonwealth, 135 Va. 524, 115 S.E. 673, 30 A.L.R. 755 (1923). Re: Commonwealth v Cody Reed Shumway Criminal Case No.: CR06-2141, Circuit Court of Virginia February12, 2007.
12. 343 U.S. 790, 72 S Ct 1002,96 L.Ed.1302 Leland v State of Oregon no 176.292 A.2d 348, 448 Pa. 299 Commonwealth of Pennsylvania v Virginia Barnes, Supreme Court of Pennsylvania, June 25, 1972.
13. Michigan Law Review, The Insanity Plea: The Uses and Abuses of the Insanity Defense, 82 MICH. L. REV.1136. 1984. Available at: https://repository.law.umich.edu/mlr/vol82/iss4/63. Accessed July 15, 2020.
14. 328NW 2d 836. (329 N.W.2d 833 (1983) State of Minnesota v. James Michael Patch No. C7-81-1043 Supreme Court of Minnesota February 18, 1983.)
15. Johnson v. Commonwealth, 135 Va. 524, 115 S.E. 673, 30 A.L.R. 755 (1923).
16. Re: Commonwealth v. Cody Reed Shumway Criminal Case No.: CR06-2141, Circuit Court Va February 12, 2007.
17. (343 U.S. 790, 72 S Ct 1002,96 L. Ed. 1302 Leland v. State of Oregon no 176.).
18. (292 A.2d 348, 448 Pa. 299 Commonwealth of Pennsylvania v. Virginia Barnes, Supreme Court of Pennsylvania, June 25, 1972.).
19. Winsdale WJ, Ross JW. The insanity plea, the uses and abuses of the insanity defense. New York: Scribner; 1983. p. 159–73.

Behavioral Health in the Lesbian, Gay, Bisexual, Transgender, Questioning, and Other as Sexual and Gender Identities Community

Johanna Greenberg, PA-C, MPAS

KEYWORDS

- LGBTQ+ • Mental illness • Suicide • Substance abuse

KEY POINTS

- Use of gender and sexual orientation identifiers should be patient selected and used during clinical encounters as well as noted in the medical record.
- Members of the LGBT+ populations have higher rates of behavioral health problems throughout their lifetimes including mood disorders, suicide risk, and substance abuse and should be screened regularly for these problems.
- Supportive community and healthcare environments for gender diverse children is important for physical and psychological development of the child.

INTRODUCTION

The lesbian, gay, bisexual, transgender, questioning, and other as sexual and gender identities (LGBTQ+) comprise a unique patient population. This population interacts with all aspects of the health care system during their lifetimes. The particular identifiers, as well as preferred pronouns, should be designated by the patient or family, in the case of young children, rather than assigned by their health care providers. A validated approach to obtaining this information from patients starting in preadolescence is the use of a *Sexual Orientation and Gender Identity (SOGI)* questionnaire (**Tables 1–3**).

Approximately 4.5% of adults (age 18 and older) in the United States identify as LGBTQ+, and in the adolescent (school grades 9–12) population, approximately 2.0% identify as gay or lesbian, 6.0% identify as bisexual, and 3.2% were not sure of their sexual identity.[1,2] It is estimated that 0.39% of the US adult population is transgender, which is defined as gender identity or expression differing in some way from their assigned sex at birth (ASAB). We should keep in mind that transgender patients

Department of Family and Preventive Medicine, University of Utah, 375 Chipeta Way, Salt Lake City, UT 84108, USA
E-mail address: Johanna.greenberg@hsc.utah.edu

Physician Assist Clin 6 (2021) 421–432
https://doi.org/10.1016/j.cpha.2021.02.005
2405-7991/21/© 2021 Elsevier Inc. All rights reserved.

physicianassistant.theclinics.com

Table 1
Sexual orientation and gender identity questionnaire

Sexual Orientation		
Do you think of yourself as:	• Straight or heterosexual • Gay or lesbian • Bisexual • Queer, pansexual, or questioning	• Something else, please specify:_____ • Don't know • Decline to answer
Gender Identity		
Do you think of yourself as:	• Male • Female • Transgender man/transman/female-to-male (FTM) • Transgender woman/transwoman/male-to-female (MTF)	• Queer gender/gender nonconforming neither exclusively male or female • Additional gender category (or other):_____ • Decline to answer
What sex was originally listed on your birth certificate?	• Male • Female • Decline to answer	

A self-reported patient survey to collect sexual orientation and gender identity information.

Table 2
An explanation of gender identity terminology

Cisgender	Gender aligns with that assigned at birth
Gender fluid	Does not align with a fixed gender
Gender nonbinary	May identify as both man and woman or outside of both of those definitions
Queergender	Reject static categories of gender and may identify as male, female, both, or neither
Transgender	Gender identity differs from sex assigned at birth

Table 3
An explanation of sexual orientation terminology

Asexual	A lack of sexual attraction toward other people
Bisexual	Attraction to more than one sex, gender, or gender identity
Gay	Attraction to people of the same gender
Lesbian	A woman who is attracted to another woman
Pansexual	Has the potential for attraction to people of any gender

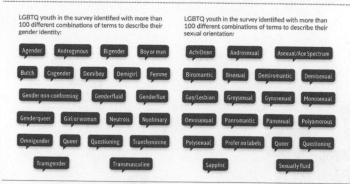

Fig. 1. Terminology used by LGBT+ youth to describe their gender identity and sexual orientation. (Reproduced with permission from The Trevor Project. National Survey on LGBTQ Youth and Mental Health 2020. The-Trevor-Project-National-Survey-Results-2020.pdf. Published 2020. Accessed 7/23/2020.)

may present with a specific gender identity or nonbinary. These patients may or may not seek to undergo medical or surgical procedures to transition gender.[3,4] A recent survey indicated that LGBTQ+ youth use a wide array of identifiers outside of LGBT, as evidenced in **Fig. 1**.[5]

As compared with their age-equivalent peers, LGBTQ+ patients experience higher rates of adverse life events related to education and employment. These can be exacerbated by a lack of federal or state policies protecting LGBTQ+ individuals from discrimination. These patients experience higher rates as victims of violent crime and of homelessness[4,6] **(Figs. 2 and 3)** This article focuses specifically on behavioral health problems that are seen at increased rates in the LGBTQ+ population. We review appropriate strategies to improve interactions between LGBTQ+ persons and their health care providers. Screening for and identifying behavioral health issues so they may be addressed will lead to improved mental health care, as well as improved general medical care.

MENTAL HEALTH DISORDERS

As compared with their non-LGBTQ+ peers, members of the LGBTQ+ community have higher rates of any mental illness (AMI) and serious mental illness (SMI) over the course of their lifetimes. The underlying causes for this are multifactorial.[7] As defined by the Diagnostic and Statistical Manual of Mental Disorders (DSM), Fourth Edition and then clarified by the DSM-5, AMI is defined as a mental, emotional, or behavioral disorder that impacts an individual's function, with impairment ranging from mild to moderate. This may include depression, anxiety, eating disorders, bipolar disorders, and/or schizophrenia. SMI is defined as an AMI that results in serious impairment in function and limits or interferes with one or more major life activities.[8]

Very early in childhood development, children begin to be able to recognize and label gender, and by the age of 5 to 6, most children are able to state their gender identity.[9] We should note that identifying with a gender identity that is different from the

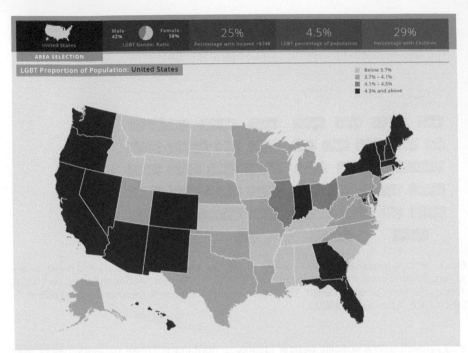

Fig. 2. The proportion of the population identifying as LGBT in the United States, further described in terms of gender identity, income status, and presence of children in the home. (Reproduced with permission from The Williams Institute, UCLA School of Law.)

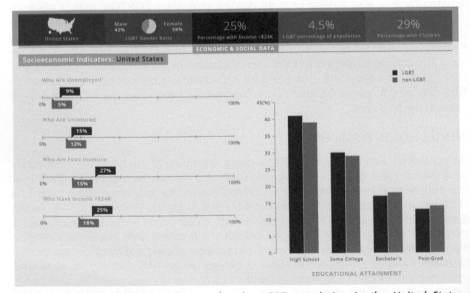

Fig. 3. Social and economic indicators for the LGBT population in the United States, including employment status, food insecurity, and level of income. (Reproduced with permission from The Williams Institute, UCLA School of Law.)

ASAB is not a pathology; however, young children can develop gender dysphoria. This is defined as significant distress or impairment in social, occupational, or other areas of function lasting for $\geq$6 months and is caused by incongruence with the individual's identified gender and ASAB.[10] Gender dysphoria should be identified and addressed in the health care setting so as to provide treatments to improve social, occupational, and educational outcomes.[11] There is compelling evidence to support the approach of educating patients and their families to use a gender-affirming approach in childhood. This approach neither discourages or encourages gender transition but rather creates an environment of family support. Children who feel accepted and supported have lower rates of behavioral health disorders.[12]

Adolescence is a time of rapid physical and psychological development, and we sometimes see the emergence of psychiatric disorders during this transition. These can include depression, anxiety, substance abuse, personality disorders, and/or psychosis.[13] Rates of these diagnoses are higher in adolescents whose parents have discouraged their gender nonconformity, increasing with additional stressors. These stressors can be physical, sexual, or emotional abuse and/or bullying encounters with their peers.[14] Gender identity and sexual orientation are some of the components of development of an individual identity that occurs during adolescence. Identifying as a gender minority itself, confers risk for stigma and discrimination that may start in childhood and continue into adolescence. This may increase when individuals experience lack of family support or overt rejection of their sexual identity. This can be particularly difficult when living in an area where there is not a large LGBTQ+ population. Individuals who are members of a gender or sexual orientation minority are more likely to experience parental physical or sexual abuse.[15] These teenagers are more likely to experience assault at school and therefore have increased absences from school due to fear. Knowledge of the aforementioned stressors can help us understand the underlying context for higher rates of SMI in the LGBTQ+ population.

In the context of health care, pre-adolescent patients' gender identity is generally described by the parents of the child. In adolescence, patients are often presented with their first opportunity to define sexual identity or to question it. This is a unique opportunity to screen for gender identity and sexual orientation. In the context of rapid biologic and social change, it is also an important time to screen for behavioral health and substance use disorders. Medical providers should use a validated screening tool to obtain information about sexual orientation and gender, a SOGI questionnaire. In addition, providers can use adolescent-specific screeners, such as the Rapid Assessment for Adolescent Preventive Services (RAAPS) or the Patient Health Questionnaire (PHQ)-9/PHQ-A to obtain additional information about socioeconomic and emotional risk factors. The adolescent patient should be allowed to complete these questionnaires in a space that is private and away from parents. Such screening tools are shown in **Figs. 4** and **5**.

Of note, the differentiation between the PHQ-9 and the PHQ-A is the addition of the last 2 questions regarding suicide risk. The addition of suicide risk questions is helpful for the screener given the higher prevalence of suicide in the LGBTQ+ community. Population surveys indicate that 40% of LGBTQ+ youth and more than 50% of transgender or nonbinary youth have considered suicide in the past year.[5] In the population at large, suicide is the third leading cause of death in people age 10 to 24 and second leading cause of death in people age 15 to 34. These risks are 4 times higher in LGBTQ+ patients.[5]

In addition, there is emerging evidence to show that in the elderly LGBTQ+ population, the risk of suicide may be on the rise due to re-closeting and social isolation.[16] Community-dwelling LGBTQ+ elders have reported stress related to fears about assisted living and nursing home settings, specifically that they will not

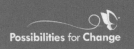

Standard RAAPS
Assessment Preview

The RAAPS assessments are comprised of 21 evidence-based questions proven to elicit honest responses from teens. The standardized, validated comprehensive assessments are available to license in a cloud-based or paper format, with three age-specific assessments available: **older child** (9-12yrs), **standard** (13-18yrs), and **young adult** (18-24yrs).

A sample question for each risk category in the RAAPS standard assessment is below.

Nutrition/Physical Activity:
Are you active after school or on weekends (walking, running, dancing, swimming, biking, playing sports) for **at least 1 hour, on at least 3 or more days each week**?

Substance Use:
In the past 3 months, have you drunk more than a few sips of alcohol (beer, wine coolers, liquor, other)?

Sexual Health:
If you have had sex, do you **always** use a condom and/or another method of birth control to prevent sexually transmitted infections and pregnancy?

Violence:
During the past month, have you been threatened, teased, or hurt by someone (on the internet, by text, or in person) causing you to feel sad, unsafe, or afraid?

Protective:
Do you have at least one adult in your life that you can talk to about any problems or worries?

Mental Health:
During the past month, did you **often** feel sad or down as though you had nothing to look forward to?

Safety:
In the past 12 months, have you driven a car while texting, drunk or high, or ridden in a car with a driver who was?

When an adolescent responds positively to any of the questions, a pre-populated health message appears upon completion of the assessment. The health messages can be used by professionals as talking points to help guide the adolescent toward positive behavior change. In the example below, the adolescent responded positively for safety risks.

HEALTH MESSAGE
Driving drunk, high, or while texting is risky and you're much more likely to be in a car crash. All of these things slow down your reaction time and makes it harder to focus while driving. You can lower your chance of an accident by following a few simple tips.

To limit the temptation to text while driving:
- Put your phone in your glove box or back seat while driving.
- Turn your phone off while driving.
- Wait until you are parked to use your phone.
- Ask a friend riding with you to text for you.

Never drive a car after using even a small amount of drugs or alcohol and avoid riding with someone who has.
- Before you go out for the night, decide who is going to be the designated driver and stick to it.
- Identify someone you can call for a ride if you find yourself in a situation that is unsafe.
- Offer to drive if you are sober.
- Find a ride from someone else.
- Call a taxicab.
- Make plans to stay the night wherever you are going.

You can make a difference in your life and the lives of your friends by making safe driving choices.

http://www.drivingsober.net/Teen-page.html
www.takethewheel.net

National Alcohol/Drug Abuse Hotline:1-800-662-HELP(4357)

Email info@Pos4Chg.org for details on how to use RAAPS to empower youth to make healthy lifelong decisions.

PHQ-9: Modified for Teens

Name: _____ Clinician: _____ Date: _____

Instructions: How often have you been bothered by each of the following symptoms during the past **two weeks?** For each symptom put an "X" in the box beneath the answer that best describes how you have been feeling.

	(0) Not At All	(1) Several Days	(2) More Than Half the Days	(3) Nearly Every Day
1. Feeling down, depressed, irritable, or hopeless?	☐	☐	☐	☐
2. Little interest or pleasure in doing things?	☐	☐	☐	☐
3. Trouble falling asleep, staying asleep, or sleeping too much?	☐	☐	☐	☐
4. Poor appetite, weight loss, or overeating?	☐	☐	☐	☐
5. Feeling tired, or having little energy?	☐	☐	☐	☐
6. Feeling bad about yourself – or feeling that you are a failure, or that you have let yourself or your family down?	☐	☐	☐	☐
7. Trouble concentrating on things like school work, reading, or watching TV?	☐	☐	☐	☐
8. Moving or speaking so slowly that other people could have noticed? Or the opposite – being so fidgety or restless that you were moving around a lot more than usual?	☐	☐	☐	☐
9. Thoughts that you would be better off dead, or of hurting yourself in some way?	☐	☐	☐	☐

In the **past year** have you felt depressed or sad most days, even if you felt okay sometimes?
[ ] Yes   [ ] No

If you are experiencing any of the problems on this form, how **difficult** have these problems made it for you to do your work, take care of things at home or get along with other people?

[ ] Not difficult at all   [ ] Somewhat difficult   [ ] Very difficult   [ ] Extremely difficult

Has there been a time in the **past month** when you have had serious thoughts about ending your life?
[ ] Yes   [ ] No

Have you **EVER**, in your WHOLE LIFE, tried to kill yourself or made a suicide attempt?
[ ] Yes   [ ] No

"If you have had thoughts that you would be better off dead or of hurting yourself in some way, please discuss this with your Health Care Clinician, go to a hospital emergency room or call 911.

Office use only: Severity score: _____

Modified with permission by the GLAD-PC team from the PHQ-9 (Spitzer, Williams, & Kroenke, 1999), Revised PHQ-A (Johnson, 2002), and the CDS (DISC Development Group, 2000)

Scoring the PHQ-9 modified for Teens

Scoring the PHQ-9 modified for teens is easy but involves thinking about several different aspects of depression.

To use the PHQ-9 as a diagnostic aid for Major Depressive Disorder:
* Questions 1 and/or 2 need to be endorsed as a "2" or "3"
* Need five or more positive symptoms (positive is defined by a "2" or "3" in questions 1-8 and by a "1", "2", or "3" in question 9).
* The functional impairment question (How difficult....) needs to be rated at least as "somewhat difficult."

To use the PHQ-9 to screen for all types of depression or other mental illness:
* All positive answers (positive is defined by a "2" or "3" in questions 1-8 and by a "1", "2", or "3" in question 9) should be followed up by interview.
* A total PHQ-9 score ≥ 10 (see below for instructions on how to obtain a total score) has a good sensitivity and specificity for MDD.

To use the PHQ-9 to aid in the diagnosis of dysthymia:
* The dysthymia question (In the past year...) should be endorsed as "yes."

To use the PHQ-9 to screen for suicide risk:
* All positive answers to question 9 as well as the two additional suicide items MUST be followed up by a clinical interview.

To use the PHQ-9 to obtain a total score and assess depressive severity:
* Add up the numbers endorsed for questions 1-9 and obtain a total score.
* See Table below:

Total Score	Depression Severity
0-4	No or Minimal depression
5-9	Mild depression
10-14	Moderate depression
15-19	Moderately severe depression
20-27	Severe depression

Fig. 5. The Patient Health Questionnaire–Teen (PHQ-9 Teen) is a 13-question (modified from 11 questions for adults) patient-completed survey that screens for depression and suicide risk. (*From* https://www.aacap.org/App_Themes/AACAP/docs/member_resources/toolbox_for_clinical_practice_and_outcomes/symptoms/GLAD-PC_PHQ-9.pdf; with permission.)

find inclusive environments. Furthermore, there is fear of dependence on health care providers, dementia, mistreatment, and isolation.[17] These concerns can provoke significant emotional stress during a time when a patient's physical health may be in decline.

SUBSTANCE USE DISORDERS

As compared with their heterosexual peers, LGBTQ+ individuals have higher rates of substance use disorders, including alcohol, tobacco, marijuana, and illicit substances. For specific groups, there are higher rates of use at certain stages throughout the lifetime. Studies have shown that substance use rates are highest in young adulthood for gay and lesbian individuals and highest in mid adulthood for bisexual men. Bisexual women experienced increased risk of substance use disorders across all age categories.[18,19]

In the adolescent population, there is a correlation between victimization at school and higher rates of substance abuse. We also see higher rates of substance use when the peer group uses/abuses substances.[20] Screening for substance use is an

Fig. 4. The RAAPS tool is a 21-question, patient-completed survey that reports domains including nutrition, physical activity, substance abuse, sexual health, violence, protective factors, and safety. (Reprinted with permission from Possibilities for Change, ©2006 The Regents of the University of Michigan, Version 8 (2020). Further reproduction or use is not permitted. For authorized use of RAAPS visit www.possibilitiesforchange.org.)

important clinical intervention that should begin in early adolescence with all of our patients, but particularly in our LGBTQ+ patients. One should realize that LGBTQ+ patients at all ages, have an increased risk for substance abuse due to underlying stressors that increase their risks. An example of an easily used screening tool to evaluate risk is the National Institute on Drug Abuse (NIDA) Quick Screen questionnaire (**Fig. 6**).

Across patient populations, there is higher risk of adverse patient outcomes when substance use or abuse co-occurs with mental illness, specifically, a higher risk for suicide.[21] Clinicians should use additional screening if they identify substance use and/or AMI during an encounter.

NIDA Quick Screen V1.0[1]

Name: .... Sex ( ) F ( ) M Age.......

Interviewer...................................... Date ....../....../......

Introduction (Please read to patient)

Hi, I'm _____, nice to meet you. If it's okay with you, I'd like to ask you a few questions that will help me give you better medical care. The questions relate to your experience with alcohol, cigarettes, and other drugs. Some of the substances we'll talk about are prescribed by a doctor (like pain medications). But I will only record those if you have taken them for reasons or in doses <u>other than prescribed</u>. I'll also ask you about illicit or illegal drug use—but only to better diagnose and treat you.

Instructions: For each substance, mark in the appropriate column. For example, if the patient has used cocaine monthly in the past year, put a mark in the "Monthly" column in the "illegal drug" row.

NIDA *Quick Screen* Question: In the past year, how often have you used the following?	Never	Once or Twice	Monthly	Weekly	Daily or Almost Daily
Alcohol • **For men, 5 or more drinks a day** • **For women, 4 or more drinks a day**					
Tobacco Products					
Prescription Drugs for Non-Medical Reasons					
Illegal Drugs					

- If the patient says **"NO"** for all drugs in the Quick Screen, reinforce abstinence. **Screening is complete.**

- If the patient says **"Yes"** to **one or more days of heavy drinking**, *patient is an at-risk drinker.* Please see NIAAA website "How to Help Patients Who Drink Too Much: A Clinical Approach" http://pubs.niaaa.nih.gov/publications/Practitioner/CliniciansGuide2005/clinicians_guide.htm, for information to **Assess, Advise, Assist, and Arrange** help for at risk drinkers or patients with alcohol use disorders

- If patient says **"Yes"** to **use of tobacco:** *Any* current tobacco use places a patient at risk. Advise *all tobacco users to quit.* For more information on smoking cessation, please see "Helping Smokers Quit: A Guide for Clinicians" http://www.ahrq.gov/clinic/tobacco/clinhlpsmksqt.htm

- If the patient says **"Yes"** to **use of illegal drugs or prescription drugs for non-medical reasons**, proceed to **Question 1** of the NIDA-Modified ASSIST.

Fig. 6. The NIDA Quick Screen tool is a 4-question survey that screens for high-risk use and/ or abuse of tobacco, alcohol, prescription medications, and illicit drugs. If the prescription or illicit drug screen is positive, an additional long form with 8 additional questions regarding drug use can be used.

The underlying reasons for higher rates of mental illness, suicide risk, and substance abuse in the LGBTQ+ population are attributed to the observed stressors referred to as the *minority stress model*.[20] This model states that when people are subjected to stigma, prejudice, and discrimination repeatedly over time and in multiple contexts, they will experience stress at a higher degree as compared with individuals who do not experience these stressors. In turn, this increases rates of mental illness as well as physical disease.[22] Conversely, we do know there are protective factors to prevent mental illness, suicidal behavior, and substance abuse. These include educational attainment, school or community engagement, higher self-esteem, and parental attachment.[23] These factors can improve outcomes in treatment of mental illness, decrease suicide rates, prevent progression of substance use to abuse, and improve socioeconomic success for members of the LGBTQ+ population.

HEALTH CARE INTERVENTIONS

Beginning in childhood, parent-child dynamics impact the physical and psychological development of the child. Theories of child-parent attachment describe different types of children.[24] The *"secure"* child has parents who are accessible and responsive to a child's needs in a sensitive manner. The *"insecure"* child does not have accessible or responsive parents and may be abused or responded to erratically. Although *secure* children are equipped to explore their environment and regulate emotions appropriately, the *insecure* child may become avoidant of parents. This child may be overly self-reliant and need to closely regulate emotions. Or, at the extreme, this child may become anxious and resistant or ambivalent about others due to a negative perception of the self. In the health care setting, we have a unique opportunity to ask questions about child attachment in the context of gender and sexuality in a safe environment. This allows us to educate both the child and the parent about skills to develop secure attachment. Furthermore, we have the opportunity to educate parents about family acceptance and support as a strong protective factor against the development of mental illness and substance abuse disorders. We can provide both the parent and the child with online resources for support, local community peer groups, and counseling service resources. This is especially valuable if the parents are struggling to understand and support a child who identifies as a sexual or gender minority.

For LGBTQ+ patients of all ages, especially into adulthood, the health care setting itself can be a stressful and anxiety-provoking environment. We have the opportunity to create a setting that is safe and welcoming for all of our patients. This can start with a basic understanding of and use of LGBTQ+ identity terminology (see **Tables 2** and **3**). In the context of providing inclusive health care, all members of the clinical team, from the front desk to nursing support to clinicians, can become educated regarding the LGBTQ+ community. Once a patient is established in the health care setting, it is important to use appropriate gender identifiers. All patients, especially our LGBTQ+ patients, should be screened for mood disorders, substance use disorders, and suicide risk. When SMI or substance abuse are identified, treatment should be initiated. This may include referrals to behavioral health or medical providers who are LGBTQ+ competent. This can be challenging because a large portion of the health care provider population has never been specifically trained regarding LGBTQ+ specific issues. In addition, there is variability between health care systems in the ability of an individual provider to identify oneself as LGBTQ+ competent.[25] Although access to LGBTQ+ competent health care is improving, there continues to be evidence that patients who are LGBTQ+ have less access to medical care than their cisgender peers.[26] Furthermore, queer, questioning, and transgender patients experience increased barriers as compared with their LGB counterparts and therefore often delay care.[26] In a survey of LGBTQ+ youth, 44% of respondents stated that in the past 12 months they wanted psychological or emotional counseling but were unable to receive it.[5] Solutions to this lack of access are moving forward and medical doctor, physician assistant, and nursing programs have begun to address LGBTQ+ topics. This education does improve knowledge, attitudes, and practices as those clinicians enter the workforce to care for patients.[27]

SUMMARY

Health care providers, whether providing medical or behavioral health care, have an opportunity to improve outcomes for LGBTQ+ patients through recognition of sexual and gender minority status. Treating patients as individuals includes using appropriate patient identifiers. Early screening and recognition of behavioral health problems with referrals to LGBTQ+ competent providers have been shown to decrease both mental and physical health issues. Educational training for health care teams with regard to LGBTQ+ care as a minority subgroup is an important part of initial and continuing medical education.

CLINICS CARE POINTS

- In a safe environment, ask patients to identify sexual orientation and gender identity using their own language.
- Screen for variations in gender identity starting in early childhood and discuss with families.
- Screen for anxiety, depression, mood disorder, suicide risk, and substance abuse in all patients, but especially in the LGBTQ+ community.
- Identify behavioral health problems and connect patients and families to management resources.
- Educate clinical staff and providers on LGBTQ+ terminology and best care practices.
- Educate students and peers on provision of improved health care for the LGBTQ+ population.

DISCLOSURE

The author has nothing to disclose.

REFERENCES

1. Newport f. In the US, estimate of LGBT population rises to 4.5%. Gallup News 2018. Available at: https://news.gallup.com/poll/234863/estimate-lgbt-population-rises. aspx. Accessed July 1, 2020.
2. Kann L, Olsen EO, McManus T, et al. Sexual identity, sex of contacts, and health related behaviors among students in grades 9-12 – United States and selected sites, 2015. MMWR Surveill Summ 2016;65(No. SS-9):1–202.
3. Meerwijk EL, Sevelius JM. Transgender population size in the United States: a meta-regression of population-based probability samples. Am J Public Health 2017;107(2):e1–8.
4. Kidd J. Mental health disparities: LGBTQ (PDF file). 2017. Available at: Mental-Health-Facts-for-LGBTQ.pdf. Accessed June 1, 2020.

5. The Trevor Project. National survey on LGBTQ youth and mental health 2020. 2020. Available at: The-Trevor-Project-National-Survey-Results-2020.pdf. Accessed July 23, 2020.

6. Morton MH, Dworsky A, Matjasko JL, et al. Prevalence and correlates of youth homelessness in the United States. J Adolesc Health 2018;62(1):14–21.

7. Medley G, Lipari RN, Bose J, et al. Sexual orientation and estimates of adult substance use and mental health: results from the 2015 national survey on drug use and health. NSDUH data review. 2016. Available at: https://www.samhsa.gov/data/. Accessed July 1, 2020.

8. National Institute of Mental Health. Mental illness. 2019. https://www.nimh.nih.gov/health/statistics/mental-illness.shtml#. Accessed August 1, 2020.

9. Martin CL, Ruble DN, Szkrybalo J. Cognitive theories of early gender development. Psychological Bulletin 2002;128(6):903–33.

10. American Psychiatric Association. Diagnostic and statistical manual of mental disorders, 5th edition Washington, DC: American Psychiatric Publishing; 2013.

11. American Psychiatric Association. Gender dysphoria. 2013. Available at: www.psychiatry.org. Accessed July 1, 2020.

12. Hill DB, Menvielle E, Sica KM, et al. An affirmative intervention for families with gender variant children: parental ratings of child mental health and gender. J Sex Marital Ther 2010;36(1):6–23.

13. Paus T, Keshavan M, Giedd JN. Why do many psychiatric disorders emerge during adolescence? Nat Rev Neurosci 2008;9(12):947–57.

14. D'Augelli AR, Grossman AH, Starks MT. Childhood gender atypicality, victimization, and PTSD among lesbian, gay, and bisexual youth. J Interpers Violence 2006;21(11):1462–82.

15. Friedman MS, Marshal MP, Guadamuz TE, et al. A meta-analysis of disparities in childhood sexual abuse, parental physical abuse, and peer victimization among sexual minority and sexual nonminority individuals. Am J Public Health 2011; 101(8):1481–94.

16. Woody I. Suicide and LGBTQ/SGL older adults. In: Diverse elders coalition blog. 2016. Available at: https://www.diverseelders.org/2016/03/20/suicide-and-lgbtqsgl-older-adults/. Accessed July 23, 2020.

17. Putney JM, Keary S, Hebert N, et al. "Fear Runs Deep": the anticipated needs of LGBT older adults in long-term care. J Gerontol Soc Work 2018;61(8):887–907.

18. Schuler MS, Rice CE, Evans-Polce RJ, et al. Disparities in substance use behaviors and disorders among adult sexual minorities by age, gender, and sexual identity. Drug Alcohol Depend 2018;189:139–46.

19. Reisner SL, Poteat T, Keatley J, et al. Global health burden and needs of transgender populations: a review. Lancet 2016;388(10042):412–36.

20. Huebner DM, Thoma BC, Neilands TB. School victimization and substance use among lesbian, gay, bisexual, and transgender adolescents. Prev Sci 2015; 16(5):734–43.

21. Suicide, facts at a glance. Available at: https://www.cdc.gov/violenceprevention/pdf/Suicide-DataSheet-a.pdf. Accessed July 23, 2020.

22. Meyer IH, Frost DM. Minority stress and the health of sexual minorities. In: Patterson CJ, D'Augelli AR, editors. Handbook of psychology and sexual orientation. Oxford: Oxford University Press; 2013. p. 252–66.

23. Kidd JD, Jackman KB, Wolff M, et al. Risk and protective factors for substance use among sexual and gender minority youth: a scoping review. Curr Addict Rep 2018;5(2):158–73.

24. Katz-Wise SL, Rosario M, Tsappis M. Lesbian, gay, bisexual, and transgender youth and family acceptance. Pediatr Clin North Am 2016;63(6):1011–25.
25. Macapagal K, Bhatia R, Greene GJ. Differences in healthcare access, use, and experiences within a community sample of racially diverse lesbian, gay, bisexual, transgender, and questioning emerging adults. LGBT Health 2016;3(6):434–42.
26. Khalili J, Leung LB, Diamant AL. Finding the perfect doctor: identifying lesbian, gay, bisexual, and transgender-competent physicians. Am J Public Health 2015;105(6):1114–9.
27. Sekoni AO, Gale NK, Manga-Atangana B, et al. The effects of educational curricula and training on LGBT-specific health issues for healthcare students and professionals: a mixed-method systematic review. J Int AIDS Soc 2017; 20(1):21624.

Where to Turn
Outpatient Services and Management

Kary Allyn Blair, BS, MBA[a,b,*]

KEYWORDS

- Deinstitutionalization • Health insurance • Mental health parity • Psychiatric care
- Outpatient services

KEY POINTS

- Deinstitutionalization has created a need to transfer psychiatric care out of inpatient hospitals into outpatient settings.
- The number of inpatient psychiatric beds (both public and private) is decreasing annually.
- There is a nationwide shortage of psychiatrists throughout the nation and many of these providers are retiring.
- Many psychiatrists do not take commercial insurance, much less Medicare or Medicaid due to inadequate reimbursement.
- Opportunities to increase the mental health workforce and increase access to care.

INTRODUCTION

Before the US public health crisis of Coronavirus Disease 2019 (COVID-19), the health care system comprised 17.7% of the gross domestic product. Health care is a $3.6 trillion per year industry, which grew exponentially with the COVID-19 crisis.[1] The federal government is the largest payer of health care services in the country through the Centers for Medicare and Medicaid Service's programs. Health care costs are growing at 3 times the rate of general inflation.[2] While spending and costs increase, access to care and quality are less than in any other industrialized nation. The United States ranks rather poorly in the primary health determinants.[3]

The author whose name is listed immediately above certifies that she has NO affiliations with or involvement in any organization or entity with any financial interest (such as honoraria; educational grants; participation in speakers' bureaus; membership, employment, consultancies, stock ownership, or other equity interest; and expert testimony or patent-licensing arrangements), or non-financial interest (such as personal or professional relationships, affiliations, knowledge or beliefs) in the subject matter or materials discussed in this article.

[a] Department of Psychiatry, Texas Tech University Health Sciences Center School of Medicine, 3601 Fourth Street, STOP 8103, Lubbock, TX 79430, USA; [b] Department of Healthcare Administration and Leadership, Texas Tech University Health Sciences Center School of Health Professions, 3601 Fourth Street, STOP 8103, Lubbock, TX 79430, USA

* Department of Psychiatry, Texas Tech University Health Sciences Center School of Medicine, 3601 Fourth Street, STOP 8103, Lubbock, TX 79430.

E-mail address: Kary.Blair@ttuhsc.edu

Physician Assist Clin 6 (2021) 433–439
https://doi.org/10.1016/j.cpha.2021.02.006
2405-7991/21/© 2021 Elsevier Inc. All rights reserved.

Mental health and substance abuse disorder treatments comprise $280.5 billion or 7% of all monies spent. The growth of spending for mental health and substance abuse disorders increases more slowly than the average annual growth of the health care system's other sectors. The annual growth has averaged 4.6%, whereas the yearly average of all health has increased by 5.8% each year.[4] Is the slower growth of spending on mental health and substance abuse disorder related to efficient care and strong cost control measures, or is it related to something far more sinister?

FACTORS LEADING TO A SHIFT FROM INPATIENT CARE TO OUTPATIENT CARE

In a movement starting in the 1950s, the United States began the process of deinstitutionalization. There has been a steady and consistent closure of inpatient beds across the country. The deinstitutionalization is in both public and private inpatient and residential beds. This trend has led to a critical shortage of inpatient and residential beds nationwide. In fact, from 1955 to 1997, more than 30% of all beds were delicensed. Between 2005 and 2010, another 25% of beds were closed. The minimum standard is to have 50 beds per 100,000 in population; however, the United States averages 11.7 beds per 100,000 in population.[5] Several factors are contributing to the movement of deinstitutionalization and the shift to outpatient care and the resultant bed shortages.

The first facilities to begin the trend of deinstitutionalization were the state hospital systems in many states. Many of these state hospitals were well over 100 years old. The facilities were in disrepair and the cost to bring them up to code was astronomical and unrealistic. In many communities, the facilities were located in rural areas.[6] This added another layer of difficulty for the facilities to attempt to hire appropriately trained staff. A crisis of too few psychiatrists is currently gripping the nation but it hits rural and community mental health systems even harder. More than half of the counties in the United States have no psychiatrist. A total of 111 million people live in a mental health professional shortage area. It is expected that by 2025, the country will have 6090 too few psychiatrists. To fuel the fire, more than 60% of psychiatrists currently practicing are older than 55 and nearing retirement. Although the Association of American Medical Colleges is working to address the shortage of psychiatrists, adding a few thousand psychiatric residents a year will not solve the workforce shortage.[7] Because of such demand, psychiatrists can choose a myriad of options and, unfortunately, state hospital systems are not a priority opportunity for many.

Private psychiatric inpatient hospitals are facing similar difficulties. Facilities are aging, and hospitals are not reinvesting in inpatient beds. Private facilities have the same recruitment woes as the state hospital systems. Hospitals and physicians recognize the reimbursement for psychiatric services is very poor. A major concern is the number of uninsured patients who need access to psychiatric care. In any given year, up to a third of patients with serious mental illness do not get access to care because of a lack of insurance coverage. Often, when in crisis, patients show up to emergency departments (EDs) for care. The Emergency Medical Treatment and Labor Act (EMTALA) ensures that patients can access care, but facilities often receive little to no compensation for the care provided. Hospitals are building new facilities without emergency rooms or inpatient psychiatric services to get around EMTALA rules.[8] As patients are released from the hospital, they cannot access outpatient care. Currently, only 55.3% of psychiatrists accept private insurance assignments, 55% accept Medicare, and only 43% Medicaid. If a patient can access an outpatient provider, very often the cost of care is far too high. It is not uncommon for patients to decompensate and then end up back in the ED and inpatient hospital because they could not be compliant with outpatient care.[9]

A consequence of lack of access to needed psychiatric care is that mentally ill patients will break laws, act out, and get arrested. The patient then enters the legal system. It is estimated that up to 50% of offenders suffer from a psychiatric condition and that treatment might have prevented their incarceration. In 44 states, jails and prisons treat more psychiatric illnesses than mental health facilities. In fact, due to access issues, New Hampshire sends nonoffenders to jail to seek psychiatric care. Of grave concern is that many of the patients in these systems do not receive the care needed. It is estimated that up to 84% are not receiving the mental health care they need. These patients would be best treated in the state hospital system, but access to these beds is shrinking quickly, as noted previously.[10]

As access shrinks, wait times in EDs extend. This has led to boarding issues within many facilities. It is incredibly disheartening that psychiatric patients remain in the ED 3.2 times longer than patients with nonpsychiatric diagnoses. Up to 60% of psychiatric patients are boarded in the ED for 24 to 48 hours. Even worse, 21% are boarded 5 days or more. The ED environment is not therapeutic for psychiatric patients, with patients receiving limited mental health care and running the risk of further decompensation.[11] The mental health population is aging, and therefore, more geriatric patients are being seen in EDs with psychiatric crises. However, due to comorbid medical conditions, these patients have a much higher acuity and require highly skilled practitioners. The geriatric population is expected to double from 2010 to 2050.[12] This adds to the risk of overwhelming the EDs, which are the safety net to psychiatric care.[13]

Patient socioeconomic status and demographics have also contributed to the shift from inpatient and residential care to outpatient care. Over the past 50 years, deinstitutionalization has been the sharpest. In the initial stages, a change in the acuity of patients required less intense care interventions; however, as time has gone on, the acuity of patient illness continues to increase. Bizarrely, this is an outcome of a growing economy and prosperity in the United States. When people have more disposable income, they can access outpatient care and receive interventions sooner to prevent an inpatient stay. However, the reverse is also true; as people lose their jobs, they lose insurance, become more disadvantaged, and both mental and physical health are often neglected. Recent trends show a drop in employer-sponsored health insurance while the issues of depression and anxiety continue to increase. Those who still have employer-based insurance realize the struggles of higher deductibles and out-of-pocket costs.[14]

Following a common financial trend in health care, mental health has developed the business strategy of using managed care to reduce spending and slow rapidly growing costs. The first goal of managed care was to create parity with the general health care counterpart.[15] However, as the wise psychiatrist, Terry McMahon, MD, once stated, "*Parity is a mirage*" (Terry C. McMahon, MD, Professor at Texas Tech University Health Sciences Center, 2020, personal communication).[16] Many health insurers excluded mental health and substance abuse treatment. This compounded the cost issue with mental health. The Affordable Care Act made attempts to improve insurance parity; however, with a decrease in patients with access to employer-based insurance and the decrease in psychiatrists accepting an assignment from insurance, this did little to increase the equality of access to care.[16] **Fig. 1** demonstrates the percentage of patients who have access to care based on their diagnosis group.

WHERE DO WE GO FROM HERE?

There are opportunities to minimize the impact of the lack of psychiatric inpatient and residential services, improve workforce issues, increase access, and to do so in an

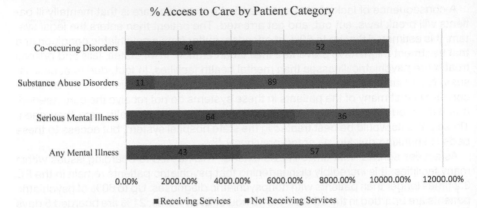

Fig. 1. Mental health disorders in US adults and access to services. (*From* Substance Abuse and Mental Health Services Administration (SAMSHA). 2017. Key Substance Use and Mental Health Indicators in the United States. Results from the 2016 National Survey and Drug Use and Health (HHS Publication No SMA 17-5044, NSDUH Series H-52).)

outpatient setting. The challenge is significant but not insurmountable. In a Centers for Disease Control and Prevention study, 45 million Americans were impacted by mental illness.[16] The average of 693 visits per 100,000 adults was to a psychiatrist compared with 397 visits per 100,000 adults for primary care (**Fig. 2**). Variances existed in rural areas where mental health visits with primary care providers outpaced psychiatrists due to a lack of specialists in rural counties. However, an annual average of 30 million mental health–related office visits were made by adults older than 18. Psychiatrists provided 55% of the care. The other 45% was supplied by either primary care or another type of specialist physician.[17]

It is evident that almost half of all mental health–related visits for adults were with a physician other than a psychiatrist; this can be exploited to increase mental health care access. A few mechanisms can help ensure primary care providers (PCPs) feel confident in treating psychiatric illness in their practices. Increasing interactions

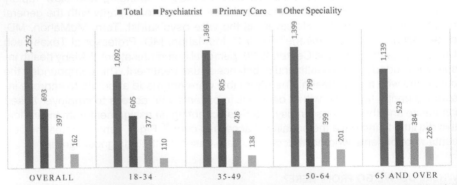

Fig. 2. Mental health–related physician office visit rates for adults aged 18 and older, by physician specialty and age group. (*From* NCHS, National Ambulatory Medical Care Survey, 2012-2014.)

between mental health experts and PCPs would expand access to many Americans who currently have none.

Physician assistants (PAs) have moved into the mental health arena. Initially, this was within the primary care offices because (as noted previously), many of the mental health patients present to their usual PCPs. Insurance often covers medical visits, but it is limited for mental health visits. PAs can diagnose and treat patients, and prescribe and manage medications while managing mental illness. Issues arose when PAs began to move into the psychiatric realm and bill under psychiatry. Although psychiatrists welcomed them, often insurance companies and regulators wanted proof of increased training. The National Commission for Certification of PAs stepped in and offered a *certificate of added quality* (CAQ), allowing PAs to treat and bill for psychiatric visits (Rodney Ho, Air Force psychiatric PA Fellowship director, 2020, personal communication).[18] Within the Department of Veterans Affairs system, one of the larger consumers of mental health services, a postgraduate physician assistant psychiatry residency is being developed to increase mental health practitioners and decrease wait times for veterans (Rodney Ho, Air Force psychiatric PA Fellowship director, 2020, personal communication).[18]

One of the first tools to assist PCPs was Project Extension for Community Healthcare Outcomes (ECHO), developed by the University of New Mexico School of Medicine. ECHO, a collaborative medical education and care management model, provides education to providers who might not be experts in the field to manage their patients' care. It is a model that takes the education and care to where the patients are. Although ECHO does not provide actual care, it does provide support and education to providers to manage the illnesses of their patients and have a safety net of support. This allows patients to have greater access to care and in a much timelier manner without increasing the cost of health care.[18]

Along the same lines, another workforce expansion model is the collaborative care model. This model has demonstrated improved patient outcomes, improved patient compliance, reduced cost, and reduced mental health care stigma. In the model, mental health care is directly integrated into primary care. The model consists of the PCP team, including a mental health care caseworker (often social worker), psychiatrist, counselor, psychologist, pharmacist, and others. The group centers the patient's care with the PCP as the point person.[19] As needed, the PCP will consult with the team regarding evidence-based patient care. The other team members make recommendations to improve outcomes. The benefit is the patient has one point of care and will not have duplication of services, diagnostics, or assessments, reducing the overall cost of care. The patient is often more engaged because it is with one provider instead of making visits to several providers. The patient forms a strong therapeutic relationship with the PCP, but gets the benefit of the team's knowledge. Access can be increased because one specialist can provide collaborative care with many PCPs.[20]

To address the increasing number of ED visits and increasing boarding times, many different options have been tried throughout the United States. The most popular is to create Psychiatric Emergency Care Centers or Diversion Centers. These centers accept psychiatric emergencies in an environment that is more appropriate for patients in crisis. The settings are not as chaotic and stress-inducing as a general ED. Patients can be assessed and stabilized and admitted to an acute unit as needed. Also, many EDs partner with a Psychiatric Extended Care Unit and a Psychiatric Assessment and Planning Unit. These units can provide short-stay beds without the fear of having to discharge a patient when observation status runs out. General EDs can partner with a psychiatric emergency room and patients can be medically cleared and go to the psychiatric ED for specialized care. In this setting, the patient is evaluated, can receive acute, intensive, but time-limited care. The psychiatrists and team can provide acute therapeutic interventions without waiting for a transfer for the general ED.[21]

The ultimate solution to improving access to psychiatric care in an outpatient setting is increased spending at the state level. When states increase funding for mental health care, it does 2 essential things. First, it reduces the stigma of mental health. Citizens will recognize the value and seek access to be treated for their mental illness without embarrassment. With 1 in 5 adults having a mental illness, decreasing stigma is critical.[22] Second, funding reduces the financial burden for the patient and his or her family. Eliminating this burden allows patients to be more compliant with their care because they can afford their medications and office visits. When patients are compliant, the cost of care goes down because the patients are more stable. Stable patients can be treated in less expensive outpatient settings, including primary care. Outpatient care allows those scarce inpatient beds to be used for the sickest patients. It also allows the revolving door to the ED and inpatient units to be slowed.[23]

SUMMARY

In the United States since the 1950s, mental health care has shifted from a focus on acute inpatient care to outpatient care. The change started to occur as state hospital systems delicensed and closed beds due to aging facilities and upkeep costs. The hospitals also suffered from poor recruitment of psychiatrists to their rural campuses. As the demand for services changed with a growing economy, many communities invested in outpatient services because patients could afford care and would be compliant. However, because of inadequate reimbursement and an aging workforce, even outpatient care began to struggle to keep up with demand. Hospital EDs went from being a safety net to being a significant supplier of psychiatric care. EDs strive to keep up with demand but have trouble transitioning patients to inpatient facilities. Solutions to the growing mental health crisis in America revolve around creating a sustainable workforce through projects such as ECHO, PAs in psychiatric care, and collaborative care models with PCPs. Additional solutions are to develop psychiatric emergency rooms and diversion centers to provide appropriate short-term acute care for patients in crisis. States must increase mental health funding to decrease stigma and decrease financial burdens allowing patients to get the care needed. This leads to more stable patients and less reliance on scarce resources.

REFERENCES

1. Centers for Medicare and Medicaid Services. 2018 NHE highlights. 2019. Available at: https://www.cms.gov/files/document/highlights.pdf. Accessed January 18, 2020.
2. Kacik A. Healthcare price growth significantly outpaces inflation. Modern Healthcare; 2018. Available at: https://www.modernhealthcare.com/article/20181025/NEWS/181029946/healthcare-price-growth-significantly-outpaces-inflation.
3. Peterson Center on Healthcare. How does the U.S. healthcare system compare to other countries?. 2019. Available at: https://www.pgpf.org/blog/2019/07/how-does-the-us-healthcare-system-compare-to-other-countries. Accessed January 18, 2020.
4. Substance Abuse and Mental Health Services Administration. Projections of national expenditures for treatment of mental and substance abuse disorders.

2010-2020. HHS publication No. SMA-14-4883. Rockville, MD: Substance Abuse and Mental Health Services Administration; 2014.

5. Medford-Davis LN, Beall RC. The changing health policy environment and behavioral health services delivery. Psychiatr Clin North Am 2017;40(3):533–40.

6. Changes to the state hospital system. Texas Health and Human Services. Available at: https://hhs.texas.gov/about-hhs/process-improvement/improving-services-texans/changes-state-hospital-system. Accessed July 31, 2020.

7. Weiner S. Addressing the escalating psychiatrist shortage. AAMC; 2018. Available at: https://www.aamc.org/news-insights/addressing-escalating-psychiatrist-shortage. Accessed July 31, 2020.

8. Misek RK, Magda AD, Margaritis S, et al. Psychiatric patient length of stay in the emergency department following closure of a public psychiatric hospital. J Emerg Med 2017;53(1):85–90.

9. Lu BY, Onoye J, Nguyen A, et al. Increased elderly utilization of psychiatric emergency resources as a reflection of the growing mental health crisis facing our aging population. Am J Geriatr Psychiatry 2017;25(6):680–1.

10. Greenwood-Ericksen MB, Kocher K. Trends in emergency department use by rural and urban populations in the United States. JAMA Netw Open 2019;2(4): e191919.

11. Manderscheid RW, Atay JE, Crider RA. Changing trends in state psychiatric hospital use from 2002 to 2005. Psychiatr Serv 2009;60(1):29–34.

12. Grafova IB, Monheit AC, Kumar R. How do changes in income, employment and health insurance affect family mental health spending? Rev Econ Househ 2020; 18(1):239–63.

13. Ayers JW, Leas EC, Johnson DC, et al. Internet searches for acute anxiety during the early stages of the COVID-19 pandemic. JAMA Intern Med 2020;e203305. https://doi.org/10.1001/jamainternmed.2020.3305.

14. Rowan K, McAlpine DD, Blewett LA. Access and cost barriers to mental health care, by insurance status, 1999-2010. Health Aff (Millwood) 2013;32(10): 1723–30.

15. Olfson M, Wang S, Wall M, et al. Trends in serious psychological distress and outpatient mental health care of US adults. JAMA Psychiatry 2019;76(2):152–61.

16. Mechanic D. Emerging trends in mental health policy and practice. Health Aff (Millwood) 1998;17(6):82–98.

17. Cherry D, Albert M, McCraig L. Mental health-related physician office visits by adults aged 18 and over: United States. NCHS Data Brief 2018;(311):1–8.

18. About ECHO. Our Story | Project ECHO. Available at: https://echo.unm.edu/about-echo/. Accessed July 31, 2020.

19. Tewksbury A, Bozymski KM, Ruekert L, et al. Development of collaborative drug therapy management and clinical pharmacy services in an outpatient psychiatric clinic. J Pharm Pract 2018;31(3):272–8.

20. Learn about the collaborative care model. Available at: https://www.psychiatry.org/psychiatrists/practice/professional-interests/integrated-care/learn. Accessed August 1, 2020.

21. Cammell P. Emergency psychiatry: a product of circumstance or a growing subspeciality field? Australas Psychiatry 2017;25(1):53–5.

22. Mental Health by the Numbers. NAMI. Available at: https://nami.org/mhstats. Accessed January 18, 2020.

23. Richardson J, Morgenstern H, Crider R, et al. The influence of state mental health perceptions and spending on an individual's use of mental health services. Soc Psychiatry Psychiatr Epidemiol 2013;48(4):673–83.

Assessment and Treatment of Psychiatric Disorders in Child and Adolescent Psychiatry

Lee I. Ascherman, MD, MPH

KEYWORDS

- Comorbidity • Multimodal treatment
- Psychotherapies (Cognitive Behavioral, Psychodynamic, Parent-Child Interactive)
- Individuals with Disabilities Education Act (IDEA) and Every Student Succeeds Act
- Biopsychosocial risk factors

KEY POINTS

- Developmental, environmental, biological and psychological forces can all contribute to symptoms and, ultimately, inform treatment design.
- Psychiatric disorders in children and adolescents encompass a remarkable variety of conditions that range in severity.
- The *Diagnostic and Statistical Manual of Mental Disorders*, 5th edition, provides a descriptive nosology, but clinicians must keep in mind that similar symptoms can have different causes, reflecting different diagnoses and treatments.
- Transitional age youth are particularly vulnerable when adult services or clinicians are not equipped to address unique challenges of transition to adulthood.
- When using medications, whenever possible, start low, advance slowly, and assess medication levels before discontinuing treatment; too rapid advancement of doses leads to side effects that deter adherence.

INTRODUCTION

Psychiatric disorders in children and adolescents encompass a remarkable variety of conditions that range in severity. Some manifest in childhood and some are seen in adults, but may first appear in childhood or adolescence. A full review of all these disorders and their treatment is beyond the scope of this article. Included for review are *Diagnostic and Statistical Manual of Mental Disorders*, 5th edition (DSM-5) diagnoses that manifest in childhood, are common in childhood, or whose morbidity warrants attention. The DSM-5 provides a descriptive nosology but clinicians must keep in mind that similar symptoms can have different causes, reflecting different diagnoses

University of Alabama at Birmingham, The Cincinnati Psychoanalytic Institute, One Office Park Suite 102, Birmingham, AL 35223, USA
E-mail address: leeascherman@gmail.com

Physician Assist Clin 6 (2021) 441–456
https://doi.org/10.1016/j.cpha.2021.03.001
2405-7991/21/© 2021 Elsevier Inc. All rights reserved.

and treatments. For example, anxiety symptoms in children can manifest with behaviors that appear as symptoms of attention deficit hyperactivity disorder. In addition, comorbidity is common in child and adolescent psychiatry.[1]

NEURODEVELOPMENTAL DISORDERS

Neurodevelopmental disorders include intellectual disability, global developmental delay, Autism spectrum disorder, attention deficit hyperactivity disorder, specific learning disorders, motor disorders including developmental coordination disorder, tic disorders, and communication disorders including language disorder, speech sound disorder, childhood-onset fluency disorder (stuttering), and social (pragmatic) communication disorder. For all of these diagnoses, early identification and intervention are essential.

Intellectual Disability

A diagnosis of intellectual disability requires "deficits in intellectual functions ... confirmed by both clinical assessment and *individualized* standardized intelligence testing and deficits in adaptive functioning that result in failure to meet developmental and sociocultural standards for personal independence and social responsibility." Severity is identified as mild, moderate, severe, or profound.[2] A youth with deficits in intellectual functioning but who has adaptive functioning does not have an intellectual disability. Neglect and hearing impairment can contribute to an erroneous diagnosis of intellectual disability and must be ruled out.

The cause of intellectual disability remains unknown for most. Nevertheless, a diagnostic assessment is essential to identify causes for which intervention can impact the course, inform genetic counseling for parents, and help parents with their adaptation and grief. The most frequent cause for intellectual disability is Down's syndrome. The second most common cause is fragile X syndrome, which is also the most common inherited intellectual disability.[3] Although most severely expressed in males, females can exhibit cognitive deficits. An intergenerational history of intellectual disability, especially among males, warrants evaluation for this disorder.

At age 3 years, children are eligible for school services under the Individuals with Disabilities Education Act, which was amended in December 2015 as Public Law 114-95, the *Every Student Succeeds Act*.[4,5] Because early intervention is critical, evaluation should not wait until age 3. By secondary school, vocational planning is crucial to facilitate a transition to adaptive adult functioning.

Communication Disorders

One of the most common special education categories used is speech and language disorders. The following guidelines highlight important considerations when a communication disorder is suspected.

- Early diagnosis and intervention are essential, especially for language delays. If a communication disorder is considered, clinicians should not wait for the upper limit of a verbal developmental milestone to be reached before initiating assessment or intervention.
- Rule out hearing impairment at the start of any assessment of a speech or language delay
- Distinguish speech from language delay. Speech refers to articulation. Language refers to all other components of communication. Although disorders of articulation can impair, language disorders are usually much more serious and warrant more complex intervention.

- Distinguish receptive from expressive language ability. Receptive language is what a child can understand when spoken to with age-appropriate language. Expressive language refers to a child's ability to communicate using spoken language.

A simple distinction between expressive and receptive language is illustrated by assessing a young child's ability to identify colors. If a child shown a red crayon is asked what color it is and cannot answer, offer the child 4 crayons of different colors and ask for the red crayon. If the child can select the red crayon, there is interference with expressive language, whereas receptive language seems to be intact.

- Distinguish shyness and inhibition from a difficulty with expressive language. Parents can provide history to help with this distinction.

Autistic Spectrum Disorder

The DSM 4 separated autistic disorder, Childhood disintegrative disorder, Asperger's disorder, and Pervasive developmental disorder not otherwise specified. These disorders were consolidated into the single diagnosis of Autistic spectrum disorder (ASD) in the DSM-5 under the category of neurodevelopmental disorders. Severities are[2]

- Level 1, requiring support;
- Level 2, requiring substantial support; and
- Level 3, requiring very substantial support.

The prevalence of ASD has increased, but research suggests that this change is not a result of increased incidence. It is explained by changes in the conceptualization of the diagnosis, the inclusion of a range of severity, a greater awareness of the diagnosis, and conflation with school categories used for service eligibility. There is actually evidence of underdiagnosis in subgroups, including those in poverty in urban centers. Unfortunately, data for rural areas does not exist, but they are also likely underrepresented. The last data available, obtained from World War II draft physicals, suggested that approximately one-third of rural draftees were disqualified by physical or mental problems. This finding actually led to government investment into training psychiatrists as an urgent need for the war effort. The rate of ASD is approximately 6.6 per 1000, is 3 to 4 more common in males than females.[6]

The full criteria for ASD can be reviewed in the DSM 5. The overarching constructs are as follows.[2]

- "*Persistent* deficits in social communication and social interaction across multiple contexts."
- "Restricted, repetitive patterns or behavior, interests, or activities."
- Symptoms must at least partially manifest in early development, not be explained by other diagnoses (ie, intellectual impairment), and must cause functional impairment.
- Specifiers include
  - With or without intellectual impairment
  - Language impairment
  - Associated with a medical or genetic condition
  - Environmental factors
  - Other neurodevelopmental, mental, or behavioral disorder
  - With or without catatonia

Assessment

There is no substitute for the clinical evaluation. Screening and diagnostic instruments specific for ASD exist. The ages and/or intellectual abilities of the children for which these instruments are designed must be considered. The Autism Diagnostic Interview–Revised for parents and the Autism Diagnostic Interview Schedule are helpful diagnostic instruments, but require significant training.[6]

Treatment

Early identification leading to early intervention is critical. Social and school interventions are as important as medications, focusing on target symptoms interfering with functioning and learning. ASD is 1 of the 13 federally recognized categories for special education under the Individuals with Disabilities Education Act.[4,5] School-based services are mandated beginning at age 3 years.[4,5] Parents and guardians often need support and guidance to advocate for their child's rights and needs as they navigate this process. They also need to access resources for children under the age of 3. The shape of psychosocial treatment and school-based interventions may vary, but most share the core strategies of behavioral interventions incorporated into applied behavioral analysis, social skills training, and strategies to promote language and communication.[6]

Pharmacologic intervention

Not all children with ASD require medication. When medication is considered, its use should be restricted to those medications with demonstrated efficacy for target symptoms or comorbid conditions. The strongest evidence for efficacy addressing aggression and irritability in children with ASD is for risperidone and aripiprazole. Antiepileptic medications have not proven effective to address these symptoms except in 1 study demonstrating moderate efficacy using sodium valproate. Selective serotonin reuptake inhibitors (SSRIs) have not proven to be helpful. There is conflicting evidence regarding the efficacy of stimulants for attention deficit hyperactivity disorder symptoms in children with ASD.[6]

Medication should never be viewed as an adequate alternative to psychosocial interventions, which include support, psychoeducation, parent guidance, behavioral interventions, social skills training, and speech and language therapy. Medication trials should focus on specific target symptoms keeping in mind that comorbid diagnoses may contribute to any presentation. Start low, advance doses slowly, and monitor for side effects. The use of atypical antipsychotics requires baseline and subsequent monitoring of lipids, cholesterol, weight, and body mass index.[7]

DEPRESSIVE DISORDERS

Depressive disorders include Disruptive mood dysregulation, Major depressive disorder, Persistent depressive disorder (dysthymia), Premenstrual dysphoric disorder, Substance/medication-induced depressive disorder, and Depressive disorder due to another medical condition. They share the symptoms of sadness, irritability, or feelings of emptiness with physical and cognitive symptoms that impact functioning.

Disruptive Mood Dysregulation Disorder

Disruptive mood dysregulation disorder was first listed as a diagnosis in the DSM 5. The impetus was a response to concerns that erratic moods in childhood were being misdiagnosed as bipolar disorder, leading to overdiagnosis and inaccurate treatment. The criteria include the following.[8]

- Severe, recurrent verbal or physical temper outbursts inconsistent with the child's developmental level, out of proportion for the situation, on average 3 or more times per week

- Between episodes, the child's mood is angry or irritable in more than 1 setting most of the day, most days
- Symptoms are of at least 12 months' duration without symptom-free periods more than 3 months
- Onset before age 10
- The diagnosis is not made before age 6 or after age 18

Major Depressive Disorder

Major depressive disorder can manifest in childhood. As children mature, their presentations can seem more like adult presentations and the rates approach those of adults. The DSM 5 criteria include depressed mood or loss of interest or pleasure most of the day, almost all days and 4 of the following:[8]

- Significant weight loss
- Insomnia or hypersomnia
- Psychomotor retardation or agitation
- Fatigue or loss of energy
- Feelings of worthlessness or excessive or inappropriate guilt
- Diminished ability to think or concentrate, or indecisiveness
- Recurrent thoughts of death or suicide with or without a plan

Symptoms are not caused by another mental disorder and manic symptoms are not part of the history. Risk factors include genetic, environmental and temperament factors.

Persistent Depressive Disorder (Dysthymia)

Because of the subtler and more enduring symptoms, persistent depressive disorder can be under-recognized. The cardinal criterion is depressed mood most of the day for most days, for at least 2 years without being symptom free for more than 2 months. In children, irritability rather than depressed mood can be evident for a duration of 1 year.

Two of the following must also be present[8]:

- Poor or excessive appetite
- Insomnia or hypersomnia
- Fatigue or low energy
- Low self-esteem
- Poor concentration or indecisiveness
- Feelings of hopelessness

Risk factors include genetic, environmental, and temperament influences.

Premenstrual Dysphoric Disorder

Premenstrual dysphoric disorder consists of symptoms during the week preceding menses that improve after menses and at least 1 of the following[8]:

- Affective lability
- Irritability or anger
- Depressed mood or significant anxiety or tension

In addition, at least 1 of the following is present:

- Diminished concentration or interest in activities
- Lack of energy

- Marked change in appetite, including overeating or cravings
- Insomnia or hypersomnia
- Feeling overwhelmed or out of control
- Physical symptoms including joint or muscle pain, weight gain, feeling bloated, and breast tenderness or swelling

Substance or Medication Induced Anxiety Disorder

The essence of this diagnosis is depressed mood and symptoms of depression attributed to a substance or medication known to be capable of creating such symptoms.

Treatment

Because of a significant response to placebo or brief supportive treatment and education, supportive psychotherapy family education and problem-solving approaches are appropriate initial interventions for mild depression. Moderate depression warrants 1 of 3 evidenced-based treatments proven to be equally effective: medication, cognitive behavioral therapy (CBT) or interpersonal therapy for adolescents.[9] Psychodynamic therapy poses challenges for empirical study because it is difficult to operationalize; however, if conducted by a skilled therapist, it can be effective. For severe or treatment-resistant depression, a combination of medication and CBT has been demonstrated to be more effective than either alone.[9]

The greatest evidence for efficacy among the SSRIs is for fluoxetine, but evidence for efficacy exists for escitalopram and sertraline. These medications can be considered when there is a failure to respond to fluoxetine or if a patient prefers these alternatives. After failure of 2 antidepressants, a third of another class such as bupropion should be considered, especially when low energy, fatigue, and psychomotor retardation are present.[9]

Children and adolescents with Disruptive mood dysregulation disorder may respond to less stimulating SSRIs such as escitalopram or sertraline. Alpha-2 adrenergic agents such as clonidine and guanfacine may address target symptoms of reactivity, impulsivity and aggression.

SUICIDE

Suicide is the second leading cause of death for ages 10 to 24 accounting for 14.7% of deaths among children age 10 to 14 and 17.6% of deaths among youth ages 15 to 24. Rates for males are greater in both age groups, although the rates for females have increased significantly in the 10 to 14 year old group. In both age groups, suicide is the second leading cause of death for Whites and Native Americans and the third leading cause of death for Hispanics. It is the fourth leading cause of death for Black children ages 10 to 14 and the third leading cause of death for Black youth ages 14 to 24. For youth ages 14 to 24, the most common methods were firearms (44.7%), suffocation (39.6%), poisoning (7.1%), and falls (3.3%). For children ages 10 to 14, the most common methods were suffocation (52.9%), firearms (40.9%), and poisoning (4.2%).[10]

The most effective public health intervention to prevent youth suicide is removal of access to firearms. Hiding or securing firearms in locked safes has proven to not be as effective as removal of firearms from the home, with tragic outcomes.[11]

Children and adolescents unable to commit to their safety should be hospitalized. Risk factors for suicide include the following.[12]

- Past and present psychiatric diagnosis, especially mood disorders and substance use disorders

- Past suicide attempts
- Acute disciplinary problems
- Adverse childhood experiences, including physical and sexual abuse
- Being the object of bullying
- Exposure to parental adverse events, including:
  - Low household income
  - Psychiatric illness in a parent
  - Suicide attempt or suicide of a parent
  - Death of a parent
  - Familial impulsive aggression
  - Chronic medical illness
  - Minority sexual orientation, especially when not accepted by family

The absence of these risk factors does not ensure there is no risk. Verbal or written contracts to not attempt suicide are not reliable, but may strengthen an alliance that can diminish risk. Parents, guardians, and some clinicians may fear that inquiring about suicidal thoughts directly will heighten risk by "planting the seed." To the contrary, it is important that there can be a direct, candid discussion of whether suicidal thoughts and plan exist and not to collude with silence about such risk.

ANXIETY DISORDERS

Anxiety disorders include Separation anxiety disorder, Selective mutism, Social anxiety disorder, Specific phobia, Panic disorder, Agoraphobia, Generalized anxiety disorder, Substance or medication induced anxiety disorder, and Anxiety disorder due to another medical disorder. Substances and medication including steroids, albuterol, pseudoephedrine, stimulants, bupropion, SSRIs and serotonin-norepinephrine reuptake inhibitors can induce anxiety symptoms. Diet supplements such as fenfluramine/phentermine or substances including marijuana, cocaine, anabolic steroids including testosterone, hallucinogens, phencyclidine, caffeine, nicotine, and withdrawal from benzodiazepines also can create or mimic anxiety.[13]

A clinical evaluation is essential and should not be replaced by any assessment instrument. Rating scales using a child self-report and parent version include The Screen for Child Anxiety Related Disorders and the Multidimensional Anxiety Scale for Children 2. The Pediatric Anxiety Rating Scale directs questions to the child or parents. The final score is based on clinician ratings from these responses. The Family Accommodation Scales-Anxiety assesses the extent to which parents change their behaviors in response to their child's anxiety.[13]

Separation Anxiety Disorder

Separation anxiety disorder is the most prevalent of anxiety disorders among children less than 12 years of age. The prevalence is 4%, decreasing to 1.6% in adolescence. More females than males are represented in community samples, but females and males present equally in clinic samples.[14] Genetic and environmental forces contribute to risks.[14] Clinical criteria include "developmentally inappropriate and excessive fear or anxiety concerning separation from" primary attachment figures manifesting with 3 of the following for at least 4 months causing significant distress or impairment in functioning[14]:

- "Recurrent excessive distress" anticipating or experiencing separation
- Fear of losing or harm coming to primary attachment figures
- Fear of an untoward event that causes separation from major attachment figures

- Reluctance or refusal to be away at school, work, or elsewhere because of the fear of separation
- Fear of being alone or without major attachment figures
- Reluctance or refusal to sleep away or sleep without being near to major attachment figures
- Recurrent nightmares pertaining to separation
- Somatic symptoms with anticipation of separation from major attachment figures

Social Anxiety Disorder (Social Phobia)

The 12-month prevalence for US children and adolescents is approximately 7% and decreases with age. Rates in the United States are higher than those elsewhere in the world.[14]

Criteria include at least 6 months of[14]:

- "Marked fear or anxiety about one or more social situations in which the individual is exposed to possible scrutiny by others"
- "Fears that he or she will act in a way or show anxiety symptoms that will be negatively evaluated"
- "Social situations almost always provoke fear or anxiety" sufficient to be "avoided or endured with intense fear or anxiety"

The fear or anxiety is out of proportion to the actual threat, causes significant distress or impairment in functioning, and is not adequately explained by a substance use, medication or a medical condition. Children can express fear or anxiety "by crying, tantrums, freezing, clinging, shrinking, or failing to speak in social situations."[12]

Selective Mutism

Selective mutism is rare, with incidence ranging from 0.03% to 1.00%. The onset is usually before age 5 years of age, but the symptoms may not be fully identified until the demands of school expose them. Clinical reports suggest many children grow out of symptoms, but comorbid social anxiety is common and these symptoms may persist. Temperament including "shyness", environment, and genetic factors have all been considered risk factors. Some parents have been observed to be overprotective or controlling. The role of genetics is supported by the large rate of comorbidity with social anxiety disorder.[14]

Criteria include the following.[14]

- Consistent failure to speak in social situations expecting speech, but able to speak in other situations
- Functional impairment of at least a month's duration other than the first month of school

Associated features include the following:

o Excessive shyness
o Fear of social embarrassment, isolation
o Negativism

PANIC DISORDER

The prevalence of panic disorder for children less than age 14 is less than 0.4%, but increases with age through adolescence, peaking in adulthood. Rates in adolescence and adulthood reach 2% to 3%. It is twice as common in females.[14]

Symptoms of panic attacks include an "abrupt surge of intense fear or intense discomfort that reaches a peak within minutes," and at least 4 of the following not better attributed to substance use, medication, a medical condition, or another mental disorder[14]:

- Palpitations
- Sweating
- Shortness of breath or choking sensation
- Chest pain
- Abdominal distress
- Dizziness or lightheadedness
- Chills or heat sensations
- Parasthesias
- Derealization or depersonalization
- Fear of losing control, "going crazy," or dying

Fear of further attacks or impairment consequent to the present attack must exist for at least 1 month.

Agoraphobia

The DSM 4 linked Agoraphobia to Panic disorder. In the DSM 5, Agoraphobia stands independent and can be diagnosed in individuals without Panic disorder. The prevalence is low in children, but by adolescence approaches the 1.7% prevalence seen in adults. Females have twice the rate of males.[14]

Symptoms include a "marked fear or anxiety" out of proportion to reality for at least 6 months involving 2 or more of the following situations:

- Public transportation
- Open or enclosed spaces
- Crowds
- Standing in lines
- Being outside the home alone
- A prominent fear of the inability to escape situations or that help will not be available should panic symptoms emerge

There must be distress or impairment of functioning. Symptoms are not better explained by substance use, medication, medical condition, or another mental condition.[14]

Specific Phobia

The criteria for specific phobia include a "marked fear or anxiety about a specific object or situation," which almost always stimulates "immediate fear or anxiety" out of proportion to the situation and sociocultural context. Physiologic arousal is usually seen, but may be evident by vasovagal responses such as fainting. The reaction must occur for at least 6 months, prompting avoidance or distressing endurance of the situation such that there is a significant impairment in functioning. A person who is frightened of bridges but can live a full life without need to cross a bridge does not have an impairment unless a needed or desired venture forces use of a bridge. The DSM 5 codes specific phobias by the specific stimulus.[14]

The 12-month community prevalence is approximately 5% for children and 16% among adolescents. The female to male ratio is 2:1, except for blood, injection, or injury phobias, which are nearly equal among males and females. There is often a precipitating trauma, such as experiencing or witnessing a dog bite, but many patients cannot identify a precipitant. Before adulthood, the intensity of symptoms often wax and wane. When symptoms persist into adulthood, they are less likely to remit. In the United States, Asians and Latinos have significantly lower rates of Specific Phobia than non-Latino Whites, African Americans, and Native Americans.[14]

Temperament and environment factors have been identified as risk factors. Genetic and physiologic factors have also been considered given family histories for animal phobias and the prominence of vasovagal syncope with blood, injection, or injury phobias.[14] Specific phobia is often the first presenting disorder among comorbid conditions, including other anxiety disorders, depression, bipolar disorder, substance use disorders, somatic symptoms and disorders, and personality disorders, "particularly dependent personality disorder."[14] Those with specific phobia are up to 60% more likely to attempt suicide than those without specific phobia disorder, but this is likely a reflection of other comorbid disorders.[14]

Treatment

The treatment of anxiety disorders includes CBT and SSRIs. Acute symptoms can be addressed with medication, but psychotherapy aimed at helping the child gain mastery of anxiety should be considered even if symptoms ameliorate with medication.[13] Elements of CBT that address anxiety symptoms include relaxation techniques, logs to enhance awareness of patterns and precipitants, graded exposure to stimuli, cognitive restructuring based on identifying thought patterns that contribute to anxiety, problem solving modeling and education, and positive reinforcement. Research provides conflicting data when CBT is compared with supportive therapy. A short-term, manualized, psychoanalytic intervention with 27 of 30 children completing treatment demonstrated a 60% remission compared with 0% among controls. Studies comparing the duration of remission in children and adolescents responding to different interventions or combinations of interventions are limited.[13]

The Child/Adolescent Anxiety Multimodal Study

The Child/Adolescent Anxiety Multimodal Study is a landmark study of treatments for anxiety disorders in youth ages 7 to 17 comparing sertraline, CBT, combined CBT and sertraline, and pill placebo. Combined treatment was superior to other interventions. There was no significant difference between CBT and sertraline alone, and pill placebo yielded the poorest outcome.[13]

OBSESSIVE-COMPULSIVE DISORDER

In the DSM 4, obsessive-compulsive disorder (OCD) was included among anxiety disorders. In the DSM 5, it is categorized distinct from anxiety disorders, as OCD and related disorders. Related disorders include Body dysmorphic disorder, Hoarding disorder, Trichotillomania (hair-pulling disorder), Excoriation disorder (skin picking), and those caused by a medical disorder.

The criteria for OCD include obsessions and/or compulsions. Obsessions are intrusive, recurrent, or persistent thoughts, urges, or images causing distress. Attempts to limit these recruit other thoughts or actions (compulsions). Religious or sexual obsessions are more common in adolescents. Fears of harm to self or loved ones are more common in children.[15]

Compulsions include repetitive actions of no rational purpose performed to contain obsessional thoughts or personal, rigid rules designed to counter distressing thoughts and/or ward off something feared. Checking, washing, sequencing, excessive praying, counting, personal words imbued with empowered meaning, and neologisms are common. Symptoms cause significant distress, time consumption, or impaired functioning.[15]

The 12-month prevalence is 1.2%. Males are more affected in childhood, but this trend reverses in adulthood to slightly more females affected than males. Up to 25% of children diagnosed have an onset by age 14; 25% of males have an onset before age 10. Without treatment, there is a low rate of remission; however, 40% may have remission by early adulthood.[15] Temperamental and environmental forces, including physical and sexual abuse and other trauma can contribute to risk. There is strong evidence for a genetic role. Children and adolescents with first-degree relatives who have OCD are 10 times more likely to develop OCD. The concordance rates for monozygotic and dizygotic twins are 0.57 and 0.22, respectively.[15]

The clinical evaluation is essential, recognizing that children are often reluctant to acknowledge obsessions and compulsions before trust is established. Parents' input also should be obtained. Screening instruments to augment clinical evaluation and monitor progress include the Children's Yale-Brown Obsessive Compulsive Scale and the Leyton Obsessional Inventory-Children's Version.[16]

Treatment

Parental guidance and psychoeducation are essential when working with children and adolescents with OCD. Medications rarely yield full remission and only 40% to 50% of drug naïve patients show partial response.[14]

CBT using graded exposure and response prevention is first line treatment in less severe cases. The Pediatric OCD Treatment Study I (POTS) demonstrated a similar response to CBT and sertraline, although responses varied by site. All sites demonstrated the superiority of CBT plus sertraline to placebo.[14] In POTS II, CBT with an SSRI was compared with SSRI alone and CBT instruction only. CBT with SSRI was significantly superior to the other 2 arms of the study. The lower rated responses, CBT instruction only and SSRI only, showed no interarm difference in response rates.[14] Fluoxetine, fluvoxamine, sertraline, paroxetine, and citalopram have been studied and found effective for OCD, although paroxetine and citalopram are not approved by the Food and Drug Administration for use in this disorder. Clomipramine, a tricyclic, was demonstrated to be more effective than SSRIs, but is not used first line given its side effect profile, including cardiac effects.[16]

SUBSTANCE-INDUCED DISORDERS

Substance-induced disorders become increasingly prevalent in adolescence. Disorders span all substances and include use, withdrawal, and intoxication. All pose acute and ongoing risk to self and others. The 12-month prevalence of alcohol use disorder is estimated to be 4.6% among youth ages 12 to 17 years of age.[17] The prevalence of opioid use disorder among those ages 12 to 17 years of age is 1.0%.[17]

Treatment of withdrawal and risks without treatment differ by substance. Alcohol and hypnotics carry the greatest risks, including death. There are shared core components of substance use treatment for all substances, but specialized interventions may be needed based on the substances involved. Comorbid psychiatric disorders are also common. Unless previously known, these disorders are difficult to diagnose before treatment of withdrawal or during intoxication. Clinicians should familiarize themselves with evaluation and treatment resources in their region. The American Academy of Pediatrics has recommended universal screening in pediatric primary settings.[18] The National Institute of Drug Abuse has recommended 2 screening instruments, the Screening to Brief Intervention and the Brief Screener for Tobacco,

Alcohol, and Other Drugs.[19,20] The CAGE and its adaption for drug use, the CAGE-AID, are instruments developed at Johns Hopkins to assess alcohol and drug use respectively.[21,22]

Post-traumatic stress disorder

In the DSM 4, Post-traumatic stress disorder (PTSD) was categorized as an anxiety disorder, but in the DSM 5 PTSD is categorized under trauma and stressor-related disorders. The criteria for PTSD differ for children younger than 6 or older than 6 years and adolescents. For children and adolescents older than the age of 6, the criteria include exposure to "actual or threatened death, serious injury, or sexual violence by direct experience of the event(s), witnessing, in person, the event(s) as it occurred to others, learning that the traumatic event(s) occurred to a close family member or friend and in the case of actual or threatened death it must be violent or accidental, or experiencing extreme or repeated exposure to aversive details of the traumatic event that is, first responders." In addition, "intrusion symptoms" linked to the event occur.

These can include:

- "Recurrent, involuntary and intrusive memories of the traumatic event(s)" that, in children older than 6 years, can be expressed through repetitive play involving aspects or themes of the trauma
- Recurrent distressing dreams related to content of or affect from the trauma; however, children younger than 6 may have distressing dreams without clear content of the event
- Dissociative reactions, including flashbacks on a spectrum of severity of loss of the present reality; in children older than 6, this can manifest as repetitive play
- "Intense or prolonged" psychological distress triggered by internal or external cues of the event or aspects of it
- Marked physiologic reactions to such cues

There is also marked avoidance of stimuli representing the event or memories of the event(s) and thoughts, feelings or external reminders of or associated with the event(s).

The individual also has "alterations in cognition or mood" as evidenced by at least 2 of the following:

- Inability to remember an important aspect of the traumatic event(s)
- "Persistent, exaggerated negative beliefs about oneself, others, or the world"
- "Persistent distorted cognitions about the cause or consequences" of the trauma, leading to blaming oneself or others
- "Persistent negative emotional state for example, fear, horror, anger, guilt, or shame"
- "Markedly diminished interest or participation in significant activities"
- Feeling detached or estranged from others
- "Persistent inability to experience positive emotions"

There is also a "marked alterations in arousal and reactivity" as manifested in 2 of the following symptoms:

- Irritable behavior and angry outbursts
- Reckless or self-destructive behavior
- Hypervigilance
- Exaggerated startle
- Diminished concentration
- Sleep disturbance

For children 6 years and younger, the object of the witnessed event or threat is often the parent or caregiver. Reenactment in play may occur without distress and physical aggression to others or tantrums may accompany heightened reactivity.[23]

By survey, 61.8% of US adolescents are estimated to be exposed to a potential traumatic event, but the lifetime prevalence of PTSD in adolescents is low at 4.7%. Females have considerably higher rates of 7.3% compared with 2.2% among males.[24]

Temperamental and genetic factors may contribute to vulnerability, in addition to environmental forces such as adverse childhood events, poverty and lack of supports, family dysfunction, parental separation, and/or death. The strength of the impact of trauma is determined by severity (dose), chronicity, degree of life threat, personal injury, interpersonal violence, and perpetration by a caregiver. Post-trauma factors improving prognosis include family support and validation of the experience and protection from stimuli representing the trauma. Dissociation at the time of trauma is also a risk factor for PTSD.[23]

Although the unexpected death of a loved one and exposure to a man-made or natural disaster are by far the most common potential traumatic events in childhood, PTSD as a consequence of these events is much lower than the rate of PTSD secondary to much less common events, including kidnapping, physical abuse by a caregiver or adult's partner, sexual abuse, and/or rape.[24] PTSD is associated with suicide ideation and attempts. Childhood abuse, a source of PTSD, is also associated with suicide.[23]

Up to 80% of those with PTSD have comorbid psychiatric disorders, including depression, bipolar disorder, anxiety disorder, and/or substance use disorder. Most young children with PTSD also have comorbid psychiatric disorders. Oppositional defiant disorder and separation anxiety disorder are most prevalent.[23] Because a diagnosis of PTSD requires a duration of more than 4 weeks, those with symptoms in the acute aftermath of trauma are diagnosed with Acute stress disorder.[23]

Assessment instruments as adjunct tools to the clinical evaluation include the Childhood Trauma Questionnaire for children 12 and above, the UCLA PTSD Reaction Index, the Trauma Symptom Checklist for Young Children, the Child Dissociative Checklist, the Adolescent Dissociative Experiences Scale, and the Child Sexual Abuse Inventory. Story based/cartoon instruments include the Darryl, the Andy/Angie Cartoon Trauma Scale and the Levonn Cartoon-Based Interview for Assessing Children's Distress.[24]

Treatment

Psychosocial intervention is the first line of treatment. The intervention with the strongest evidence-based support is trauma-based CBT for children aged 3 to 18 years. It includes psychoeducation, relaxation skills, affective modulation skills, cognitive coping and processing, development of a trauma narrative, in vivo mastery of trauma reminders, conjoint child–parent sessions focusing on the child's trauma narrative and family issues, and enhancement of the child's safety and development.[24]

Although there is evidence for SSRIs being effective in the treatment of adult PTSD, there is no such evidence for children and adolescents. Two studies of sertraline showed no benefit over placebo.[24] Small sample studies have suggested benefits with quetiapine, clonidine, and guanfacine. Propranolol has been suggested as helpful for hyperarousal and flashbacks. There has also been a suggestion that D-cycloserine, an NMDA agonist, can be helpful toward fear extinction and may be beneficial in other anxiety disorders in children.

About 20% of children and adolescents continue to meet the criteria for PTSD following trauma-based CBT. Because no medication is approved by the US Food and Drug Administration for PTSD in children and adolescents, medication trials should address target symptoms and comorbid disorders.[24]

SUMMARY

Those who work with children and adolescents with mental health vulnerabilities encounter an incredibly wide range of disorders that demand attention to biological, social, and psychological forces. Clinicians are privileged with entrée to deeply personal issues requiring empathy and tact. Tolerance of ambiguity is also needed, recognizing that important aspects of the history may not be easily discovered without support and patience. In addition, for many families, fear of stigma, though unfortunate, is present. Some youth will present with needs that can be easily and quickly addressed, whereas others will have much more complex needs and will require long-term treatment and support.

The key elements of skilled practice include the following.

- Attention to social, environmental, and psychological forces as well as biological.
- Multimodal treatment ie, medication and psychotherapy is usually more effective than a single modality, especially in more moderate to severe presentations.
- Education about aspects of diagnosis and treatment, including psychoeducation and/or parent guidance, is essential.
- Before arriving at diagnostic conclusions, keep in mind that symptoms of distinct diagnoses can overlap and comorbidity is common.
- Continuity of clinicians and treatment settings is ideal and should be included in the design of clinics.
- Transitional age youth are particularly vulnerable when adult services or clinicians are not equipped to address the unique aspects of young adults. Whenever possible, maintain flexibility continuing with patients beyond age 18 or, if not possible, until adequate resources are available.
- When using medications, whenever possible start low, advance slowly, and when available, assess medication levels before discontinuing treatment. Too rapid advancement of dosages leads to side effects that deter adherence.
- When multiple medications are needed owing to refractory symptoms, add before removing the one in question so that optimal assessment of each medication's efficacy can occur.
- Avoid rapid discontinuation of medications for which there is a possibility of withdrawal symptoms.
- Be aware of your own reactions to patients and caretakers or prejudices.
- Advocate for seeing patients as frequently and for as long a duration as possible for adequate monitoring and depth of communication.
- With written consent, advocate for patients and families to schools and agencies in the community. Avoid delegating communication to those who know the patient less well.
- At the same time, guard confidentiality by not sharing details about an individual or family member, verbally or in writing, that is not relevant to any immediate issue. Avoid sending summary documents that share more than the receiving party need to know, especially documents that include family issues and history that breach other's privacy. Clarify what the receiving party actually needs, and consider sending a summary letter that includes this, rather than a summary document that reveals far more than necessary.
- Err in the direction of protecting a child in situations when there is ambiguity regarding informing child protective services or when recommending hospitalization.
- When reporting abuse or neglect, strive to be open with families about this. Consider offering that parents or guardians be in the room or make the call

with you present. This practice can strengthen the long-term alliance and prevent suspicion about what was said, as well as demonstrate that the family is engaged in treatment.

- Always strongly advocate that all firearms be removed from the home, consistent with the American Academy of Pediatrics and Academy of Child and Adolescent Psychiatry recommendations.
- Be as aware as possible of your own sensitivities, reactions, and prejudices to manage them and minimize their interference in care.
- Remain open minded to diagnostic questions and evolving courses. Avoid reductionist conclusions that foreclose on new considerations.
- Seek consultation when facing challenging situations; welcome input from others.

Those working in child and adolescent mental health will discover a challenging practice demanding sensitivity, introspection, and awareness of self. Communication skills are required as is the ability to consider the relative contributions from biological, psychological, social and environmental forces in order to design effective treatment. The rewards are those that come with helping children and families through a wide variety of painful and difficult challenges as development unfolds. Some may provide more immediate satisfaction, akin to Anna Freud's imagery of placing a toy train back on its tracks so that development is free to proceed. Others will require long-term assistance and repeated help to get back on track. In either situation, clinicians fortunate enough to assist these children are rewarded with the satisfaction of knowing they offer unique knowledge and skills to help the children and adolescents they meet suffer less and move forward at the leading edge of their abilities.

DISCLOSURE

The author has nothing to disclose.

REFERENCES

1. Fombonne E. Epidemiology. In: Martin A, Bloch MH, Volkmar FR, editors. Lewis's child and adolescent psychiatry. 5th edition; 2018. p. 220. Philadelphia, PA.
2. Neurodevelopmental disorders, diagnostic and statistical manual of mental disorders (DSM-5). 5th edition. p. 33. Washington, DC. 50-51.
3. Tomasi S, Lennington JB, Leckman JF, et al. Molecular Basis of Select Childhood Psychiatric Disorders. In: Martin A, Bloch MH, Volkmar FR, editors. Lewis's child and adolescent psychiatry. 5th edition; 2018. p. 267. Philadelphia, PA.
4. Individuals with Disabilities Education Act (IDEA), original Pub.L. 105-17, revision Pub.L.101-476 20 U.S.C. Ch. 33: 2004/Code of Federal Regulations 34CFR Part 300 and 301 August 2006.
5. Every student Succeeds act (ESSA), 20 U.S.C. § 6301. Available at: https://www.congress.gov/bill/114th-congress/senate-bill/1177.
6. Volkmar FR, Van Schalkwyk GI, Van Der Wyk B. Autism spectrum disorders. In: Martin A, Bloch MH, Volkmar FR, editors. Lewis's child and adolescent psychiatry. 5th edition; 2018. p. 423. Philadelphia, PA. 427, 429-431.
7. Birmaher B, Goldstein T, Axelson DA, et al. Bipolar spectrum disorders. In: Martin A, Bloch MH, Volkmar FR, editors. Lewis's child and adolescent psychiatry. 5th edition; 2018. p. 495. Philadelphia, PA.
8. Depressive disorders, diagnostic and statistical manual of mental disorders (DSM-5). 5th edition. p. 156. Washington, DC. 160-161, 168-169, 171-172.

9. Brent DA. Depressive disorders. In: Martin A, Bloch MH, Volkmar FR, editors. Lewis's child and adolescent psychiatry. 5th edition; 2018. p. 476–8. Philadelphia, PA.
10. Pfeffer CR. Child and adolescent suicidal behavior. In: Martin A, Bloch MH, Volkmar FR, editors. Lewis's child and adolescent psychiatry. 5th edition; 2018. p. 500. Philadelphia, PA.
11. American Academy of child and adolescent psychiatry facts for families, No. 37.
12. Pfeffer CR. Child and adolescent suicidal behavior. In: Martin A, Bloch MH, Volkmar FR, editors. Lewis's child and adolescent psychiatry. 5th edition; 2018. p. 501–4. Philadelphia, PA.
13. Taylor JH, Lebowitz ER, Silverman WK. Anxiety disorders. In: Martin A, Bloch MH, Volkmar FR, editors. Lewis's child and adolescent psychiatry. 5th edition; 2018. p. 513-4. Philadelphia, PA. 514-515.
14. Anxiety disorders *diagnostic and statistical Manual of mental disorders (DSM-5)*. 5th edition. p. 190–3. Washington, DC. 195-198, 200, 202-203, 208-210, 217-219.
15. Obsessive compulsive disorder *diagnostic and statistical manual of mental disorders (DSM-5)*. 5th edition. p. 237–40. Washington, DC.
16. Towbin KE, Riddle MA. Obsessive compulsive disorder. In: Martin A, Bloch MH, Volkmar FR, editors. Lewis's child and adolescent psychiatry. 5th edition; 2018. p. 523–6. Philadelphia, PA.
17. Substance use disorders *diagnostic and statistical Manual of mental disorders (DSM-5)*. 5th edition. p. 493. Washington, DC. 543.
18. American Academy of Pediatrics, Substance use screening and brief intervention for youth. Available at: www.aap.org.
19. Screening to Brief Intervention (S2BI). Available at: www.drugabuse.gov/ast/s2bi/.
20. Brief Screener for Tobacco, Alcohol, and other Drugs. Available at: www.drugabuse.gov/ast/bstad/.
21. Available at: pubs.niaaa.nih.gov/publications/arh28-2/78-79.
22. Available at: www.ncbi.nlm.nih.gov/pmc/articles/PMC5094106/.
23. Trauma- and stressor related disorders *diagnostic and statistical manual of mental disorders (DSM-5)*. 5th edition. p. 271–4. Washington, DC. 277, 278, 280-281.
24. Hoover D, Kaufman J. Posttraumatic stress disorder. In: Martin A, Bloch MH, Volkmar FR, editors. Lewis's child and adolescent psychiatry. 5th edition; 2018. p. 654. Philadelphia, PA. 656-657.

Seasons and Seasonings of the Older Years
Psychiatric Issues in the Elderly

Jay C. Somers, MS, PA-C, DFAAPA[a],*,
Charlene M. Morris, MPAS, PA-C, DFAAPA[b]

KEYWORDS

- Geriatric • Geriatric psychiatry • Dementia • Elderly depression
- Elderly health disparitry

KEY POINTS

- Geriatric mental health is a worsening problem and requires identification and intervention.
- Dementia is intertwined in the geriatric mental health paradigm. Dementia my occur separately or comorbid with other mental health conditions.
- Polypharmacy: narcotic and non-narcotic modalities often are associated, if not causative of, geriatric mental health maladies.
- Pain worsens mental health problems, and hurt can cause mental decompensation when unrelenting and not treated.
- Abuse, isolation, and loneliness are issues that are more identified recently as having an impact on mental health, especially in those over 65.

INTRODUCTION

The US population is aging. With aging come challenges, responsibilities, and issues of personal, societal, and political importance for the medical community. Geriatric medicine is practiced in uncharted territory, as people are living longer than they ever have in history. By 2035, fully 20% of those living in the United States will be over age 65. Looking further down the road, in 2050, 10 million of the elderly population will have achieved the age of 90 and above, presenting even more challenges. Mental health, including depression, anxiety, and often dementia, is inextricably connected to physical health and aging. These conditions have come to the forefront both in visibility and acceptance thanks to both recognizable older faces and the

[a] 8545 West Warm Springs Road, Suite A-4 #210, Las Vegas, NV 89113, USA; [b] Louisville, KY, USA
* Corresponding author.
E-mail address: JCSomersPAC@gmail.com

Physician Assist Clin 6 (2021) 457–466
https://doi.org/10.1016/j.cpha.2021.02.007
2405-7991/21/© 2021 Elsevier Inc. All rights reserved.

commonality of conditions. Optimizing mental health and dealing with mental disease not only in the at-home elderly population but also in skilled nursing facilities and assisted living facilities have become the focus of discussions for both the medical community and society.

AGING AND DECLINING HEALTH

For purposes of this article, *older* is defined utilizing the established Medicare definition as 65 years old. With age, services may be necessary to sustain a person's declining physical and mental health and the conditions surrounding what is considered normal aging. Often, practitioners in medicine have priorities of prolonging life and avoiding medical-legal issues; thus, safety and protocols are stressed to prevent damaging events, such as medication errors, falls, and physical injury.[1] In contrast, when asked, patients request independence, comfort, and food choices. They want to avoid suffering, maintain mental acuity, and achieve a sense that their life has completed its purpose.[1] It is incumbent on practitioners to take the path of preferences from patients and respect their wishes and designated desires.

HEALTH DISPARITIES IN THE ELDERLY

The mental health of the elderly deserves the same attention as their physical health.[2] Approximately 20% of Americans over age 55 have some type of mental health concern whereas recent Centers for Disease Control and Prevention (CDC) data show that older men have the highest rate of suicide of any group.[2] The mental health effects of loneliness, depression, insomnia, and/or cognitive impairment highlight that the mental health issues of elderly adults face enormous obstacles to being identified and treated appropriately. The elderly also experience worse clinical outcomes.[3,4] The common issues of aging (ie, decreased ambulation, vision, and/or hearing deficits and/or decreased cognition) mean the elderly may be overlooked when evaluating for mental health issues.

Health disparities permeate many aspects of American culture, including care for the older population. This is true across measures of disability, disease, and personally assessed feeling of well-being.[5] When compared with elderly whites, elderly Latinos have higher rates of diabetes and disabilities whereas elderly African Americans have more chronic health conditions.[5] Even after controlling for variations in the economic situation and the higher incidence of chronic health conditions, the percentage of African Americans receiving mental health care is only half that of whites.[6] From a sociologic point of view, African American and Hispanic populations are more reluctant to see a mental health specialist than other groups.[6] Hispanics and African Americans have decreased rates of psychotherapy and pharmacotherapy in mental health settings than do whites.[6] The elderly themselves, as a broader population, represent a minority group that often is subject to discrimination, with differences in access, screening, or treatments based solely on their age. Even among elderly non-Hispanic white Americans, the impact of income and gender cause health status to dramatically differ.[5]

Along with the substantially growing subpopulation of elderly in the United States, African American, Hispanic, and Asian populations are increasing as a percentage of the older total population. Some of this is due to an increase in life spans but also an increase in the minority makeup of the general population.[7] There is a need for research into the health in elderly minority populations, looking at subpopulations to better understand the cultural, historical, and sociopolitical backgrounds of many older minority adults.[8]

It is important to evaluate health literacy, including numeracy, in treating the elderly to translate known physical and mental health information into useable, accessible, and actionable guidelines for patients and frontline caregivers.[9] As patients age, impairment is seen in the ability to create a "single memory structure" integrating both the item to remember and the source.[10] The issues of vision, deafness, decreased ambulation, memory loss, and increased information needed to navigate the health care system, overlaid with provider interactions via computerized contact, mean that the elderly often are left behind.[11]

ABUSE, ISOLATION, AND LONELINESS

Elder abuse is insidious and may be subtle in its presentation. There are multiple types of elder abuse, including neglect, sexual exploitation, and financial abuse. Women are more likely to be affected.[12] Subdued reactions of the patient to family members and caretakers may be a sign. Without caregivers present, cautious conversation and interviewing may reveal patient concerns. Physical signs include bruises, skin tears or lesions, weight changes, and more obvious indicators of urine or fecal odors with hygiene changes.[13] The social isolation that often is experienced by the elderly puts many at higher risk for domestic violence, depression, and harm.[14]

Delayed medical and mental health care, along with neglect and abuse, are only some of the many conditions affecting the elderly. Social relationships are vital to well-being, and research consistently has shown a strong correlation between perceived feelings of loneliness and worsening physical and mental health outcomes.[15] Social isolation and loneliness often are ignored in medical evaluations despite having a high correlation to mortality.

According to the US Census Bureau, the number of American households with just 1 person has been rising over the past 50 years and in 2019 topped 28%.[16] Furthermore, between 1990 and 2010, there has been a 3-fold increase in the number of Americans who reported having no close confidant in their social circle.[17] Loneliness and social isolation have been persistent mental health problems for Americans for many years. These problems disproportionately affect middle-aged and elderly Americans due to factors, such as grown children moving out of the house, greater geographic dispersal of close family throughout the country, retirement or disability from work, and life partner death or separation. Social isolation is an objective measure regarding the number of social connections kept and interactions that occur within a social circle. Loneliness, however, is a subjective assessment measuring 2 unmet needs: social support and companionship.[18]

These 2 components of loneliness (social support and companionship) have been correlated significantly with increased heart disease risk.[15,18] Cumulative empiric evidence across 148 independent studies suggest that individual experiences within various social relationships significantly predict mortality.[17] Social isolation and loneliness have a well-established mortality risk that is comparable to daily cigarette smoking and that exceeds the influence of physical inactivity and obesity.[17] For the elderly and infirm, often demographic disparities, such as race, ethnic origins, financial issues, and cultural differences, make them some of the most vulnerable.[19]

DEMENTIA, DEPRESSION, AND COMORBIDITIES

Aging changes how the mind works. Recall is slower and behavior can be dysfunctional progressing to dangerous for the patient or others. Basic screening and direct referral for definitive testing and evaluations often are reasonable and prudent actions.[20,21] Testing may include the physical (history/physical, laboratory studies, and imaging) along with the psychological (screening for dementia and/or depression). Men over age 65, especially those with multiple comorbid diseases, are at high risk for self-harm.[22] Much of this is related to loss, including death or divorce of their partner, failing health, changes in finances, and/or decreased engagement in their community.[22] The recent COVID-19 restraints highlighted and exacerbated a growing problem with isolation and the feeling of disconnection and disenfranchisement from family, friends, and community. These feelings can result in suicidal thoughts and, too often, the act itself.[23]

A grief reaction from a patient who is declining and aging is not unexpected. There is an expanding list of comorbid conditions directly associated with depression. Although the common ones are well-known (diabetes, Parkinson disease and/or post-myocardial infarction), there are less commonly identified conditions. One of these is inflammatory bowel disease with changes in the gut and microbiome linked to dementia and depression.[24]

Recent clinical studies have shown that hydration affects cognitive performance, in particular visual attention and mood.[25] Dehydration is a common cause of electrolyte imbalances from either inadequate fluid intake or higher metabolic needs.[26] An emerging theory states that long-term dehydration is one of the primary mechanisms behind the development of diabetes, hypertension, obesity, and several forms of dementia, including Alzheimer disease.[25] This can be a bidirectional issue because malnutrition and dehydration, which frequently are experienced by patients with dementia, can lead to hospitalization and decreased quality of life.[25] Visual impairment, disability, incontinence, speech issues, medications, and swallowing issues can affect fluid intake.

The physiologic and hormonal inability to regulate internal fluid status leading to dehydration is one of the earliest signs of neuronal dysfunction, Alzheimer disease, and/or brain atrophy.[25] Because total body water decreases with age and body mass index (BMI) increases with age, the elderly and/or obese patients may be chronically dehydrated.[25] Dehydration has been significantly correlated with worsening dementia as well as predisposing patients to acute delirium.[26] Considering the role of abnormal fluid status in the assessment of acutely worsening dementia or acute delirium is vital.

Adequate nutritional intake is an essential consideration in the elderly; however, the United States is not facing a massive malnutrition problem but quite the opposite. The CDC reports the age-adjusted prevalence of obesity (BMI >30) among those aged greater than 60 years old is 43.3%.[27] The incidence of obesity and severe obesity (BMI >40) is increasing for both male and female older adults.[27] The obesity crisis is leading to an increase in comorbidities, including depression and mental illness.[28] Although malnutrition may be less of a concern in the general population, it can be an issue with the financially insecure older adult.

The role of sleep cannot be understated. Each person has a unique sleep requirement, dependent on genetics, gender, age, previous sleep patterns, and physiologic factors.[29] Lack of sleep and poor sleep quality have been tied to mental health issues, including depression and anxiety. The incidence of sleep issues increases with age from 33% for those below age 65 to 50% of those over age 65.[30] Although many patients believe reduced sleep quality and quantity are normal processes of aging, poor sleep in the elderly often is related to psychiatric, medical, and primary sleep disorders.[31,32] Poor sleep can lead to deficits in memory, concentration, attention, and driving ability and can increase fall risk, depression, suicide and Alzheimer disease.[33] Sleep and depression are intertwined because depression affects both sleep onset and maintenance but a restoration of sleep correlates with a decreased severity of depression.[34]

Major depressive disorder can disrupt sleep maintenance, leading to early morning awakenings.[35] The frequency of sleep disorders may be as high as 30% in vascular dementia and Alzheimer disease and up to 40% in dementia related to Parkinson disease and Huntington disease.[35] A first major depressive episode in a person over age 65 has been identified as a significant independent risk factor for developing dementia.[35] In this patient population, it can be challenging to distinguish dementia plus a major depressive episode versus each one separately. Major depressive disorder generally develops over weeks to months and is, importantly, a new impairment for the patient. Conversely, dementia alone may develop insidiously over months or years and generally is slow in symptom progression. If both are suspected at the time of evaluation, it often is necessary for the depressive episode to improve before dementia can be definitively diagnosed.[35]

Numerous medical issues in the elderly that can affect sleep include sleep apnea (increased BMI), reduced cognitive capacity, dementia, restless legs (circulatory issues), arthritis (pain), nocturia, gastroesophageal reflux, paroxysmal nocturnal dyspnea, and changes in the circadian rhythm that come with age.[36] The circadian rhythm disorder found most commonly in the elderly is advanced sleep-wake phase disorder, causing patients to feel excessively tired at 5:00 PM to 6:00 PM and then waking at 2:00 AM to 3:00 AM .[37,38] Chronic depression is a major causative factor in circadian rhythm disruptive sleep. Depression is more frequent in the elderly and is correlated with underlying brain changes, increasing the risk of dementia.[39] Older women may be more sensitive to the impact of aging on sleep and at higher risk for sleep disturbance and thus have increased risk for depressive symptoms, dementia, and general cognitive decline.[40] Nonpharmacologic interventions, such as light therapy, cognitive-behavior therapy, exercise, social activities, and/or sleep routines, may help with sleep.[40–42]

PAIN, POLYPHARMACY, AND THE PSYCHIATRIC OVERLAP

Polypharmacy may present as mental status changes. When examining the causes of deterioration of the mental status of patients, one of the first considerations is to look at medications and their interactions. One issue is opiates, often abused drugs, which, if taken in combination with benzodiazepines, can mimic medical and mental deterioration.

Pain was renamed the fifth vital sign in 1995, and it became a usual practice to treat pain with drugs that often resulted in iatrogenic addiction as well as depression and paradoxically worsened existing anxiety.[43] With the advent of the dramatic rise of addiction and deaths, in 2016, the American Medical Association voted to stop treating pain as the fifth vital sign, hoping to decrease addiction rates.[43] The Beers Criteria discusses inappropriate dosing for the older adult along with issues in combination medications and drug-drug interactions.[44]

Often over-the-counter (OTC) or complementary alternative medications (CAMs) can assist in managing pain in the elderly.[45] They can be started with music, tai chi, and/or yoga, with OTC treatments, such as transepidermal neurostimulation, ice/heat, and/or biofeedback.[46–50] Many CAM medications, such as ginkgo biloba or turmeric, after screening for polypharmacy and drug/drug interactions, can be used safely for pain in the elderly.[45] Topical medications are underutilized and can include menthol creams, OTC lidocaine patches, topical lidocaine cream, diclofenac gel (safe for the kidney patient if applied appropriately), capsaicin cream, and/or amitriptyline with ketamine cream.[51]

An interesting outgrowth of the legalization of medical marijuana in many states has been the increased use of cannabis in the elderly. Marijuana is the most commonly used illicit drug among older adults and the greatest increase is seen in patients ages 50 and older.[52] States that release data by age group show the largest growth in medical marijuana cards is the greater than 60-years-old category. This is true even with states that allow for recreational use of marijuana. Medical Marijuana, usually in oral or sublingual formulas, is considered to be safer than many pain medications in the elderly population[53,54] Often practitioners do not question older patients on their use of marijuana. Marijuana can affect central nervous system cognition and is a known cause of metabolic acidosis and thus is an important data point to collect.

THE INTERSECTION OF CORONAVIRUS AND THE ELDERLY

The physical health and financial costs of the 2020 coronavirus (COVID-19) pandemic resulted in emotional responses, including general feelings of overwhelming anxiety, helplessness, and despair, in response to circumstances over which most had minimal control.[55] The required quarantine and physical distancing measures directly affected the elderly. Because COVID-19 mortality was higher in those greater than age 85, aggressive isolation procedures were implemented in many retirement communities, nursing homes, and elderly living facilities.[56] This, in turn, caused increased issues with loneliness and depression.[57] Social relationships are vital to well-being, and research consistently has shown a strong correlation between perceived feelings of loneliness and worsening physical and mental health outcomes. Social isolation and loneliness often are ignored in medical evaluations, despite having a high correlation with mortality.[16,58]

In addition to its effect on mental health, COVID-19 had profound effects on medical health care delivery and access. Patients were more likely to have skipped or postponed medical care, and this proportionately affected those with chronic conditions. Many providers turned to phone visits or telehealth.[59] This required Internet access and skills that many elderly patients found challenging.[60,61] The full ramifications and outcomes of the COVID-19 response and sequela on the mental and physical health of the elderly is an unfolding story and will be for many years.

LIVING TO 90 AND BEYOND: WHO WANTS TO GO?

Grow old along with me. The best is yet to be!

—Robert Browning

Growing older largely is uncharted territory in the United States. By 2050, almost 10 million people will be nonagenarians. Dementia plagues approximately 50% of those living to this super-age of 90-plus.[62] If not dementia, amyloid-type Alzheimer often is found in the brains at autopsy, typically in direct correlation with the decline of physical health and abilities to perform self-care.

Mental health and the older adult will continue to be closely correlated. Whether mental health changes are due to medication, aging, or depression, the need for mental health experts in gerontology who can distinguish the cause is acute.[63] It is estimated that 15% of adults over the age of 60 have a mental health disorder, and the rate of dementia is expected to triple in the next 30 years.[64]

For this group of patients, lifestyle changes have been very effective. The changes encompass a variety of forms, including gardening, pets, weight loss, exercise or increased activity, adequate housing, security, and social programs.[64–67] It is incumbent upon practitioners to care for this high-risk population. After all, we will all be there in a very few years.

CLINICS CARE POINTS

- Mental health issues in the elderly are often overlooked due to the more common issues of aging: decreased ambulation, decreased vision, and hearing.

- Ask your patients about marijuana use as the largest group with medical marijuana cards are the 60 years old.

- Elder abuse is more common than you think; be sure to make time to talk to your patients without the caregiver in the room.

- Fluid status issues in the elderly can present as confusion. Fluid issues may be a side effect of medication or of the older adult's fear of incontinence.

- Consider the importance of quality sleep and nonpharmacological approaches to pain control as these two factors have significant influence over mental health concerns.

DISCLOSURE

None: C.M. Morris; none: J.C. Somers. Both authors were responsible for the research, development and writing of the article.

REFERENCES

1. Gwande A. Being mortal, medicine, and what matters in the end. Stuttgart (Germany): Macmillan Books, Holtzbrinck Publishing Group; 2014.
2. Centers for Disease Control and Prevention. The state of mental health and aging in America 2018. Available at: https://www.cdc.gov/aging/pdf/mental_health.pdf?fbclid=IwAR2K-CtioOreiGYNe-FZbCkLWQ54BYfOF61a6ON36-xYue2SASt71qlzSeU. Accessed June 2, 2020.
3. Levine D. Why mental illness is so hard to spot in seniors. 2018. Available at: https://health.usnews.com/health-care/patient-advice/articles/2018-06-15/why-mental-illness-is-so-hard-to-spot-in-seniors. Accessed June 14, 2020.
4. Jimenez DE, Cook B, Bartels SJ, et al. Disparities in mental health service use of racial and ethnic minority elderly adults. J Am Geriatr Soc 2013;61(1):18–25.
5. Dilworth-Anderson P, Pierre G, Hilliard TS. Social justice, health disparities, and culture in the care of the elderly. J Law Med Ethics 2012;40(1):26–32.
6. Dobalian A, Rivers PA. Racial and ethnic disparities in the use of mental health services. J Behav Health Serv Res 2008;35(2):128–41.
7. United States Census Bureau. New census bureau report analyzes US population projections. 2015. Available at: https://www.census.gov/newsroom/press-releases/2015/cb15-tps16.html. Accessed June 15, 2020.
8. Thorpe RJ Jr, Whitfield KE. Advancing minority aging research. Res Aging 2017;39(4):471–5.
9. Picetti D, Foster S, Pangle AK, et al. Hydration health literacy in the elderly. Nutr Healthy Aging 2017;4(3):227–37.
10. Ansburg PI, Heiss CJ. Potential Paradoxical Effects of Myth-Busting as a Nutrition Education Strategy for Older Adults. Am J Health Education 2012;43(1):31–7. Available at: http://search.ebscohost.com/login.aspx?direct=true&AuthType=shib&db=s3h&AN=70862090&site=eds-live. Accessed June 28, 2020.
11. Serper M, Patzer RE, Curtis LM, et al. Health literacy, cognitive ability, and functional health status among older adults. Health Serv Res 2014;49(4):1249–67.

12. Social isolation, loneliness in older people pose health risks. Available at: https://www.nia.nih.gov/news/social-isolation-loneliness-older-people-pose-health-risks. Accessed June 29, 2020.

13. COVID 19 and Social Isolation. Available at: https://journal.ahima.org/covid-19-and-social-isolation-puts-elderly-at-risk-for-loneliness/. Accessed June 29, 2020.

14. Elder Abuse. Available at: https://www.nia.nih.gov/health/elder-abuse. Accessed June 29, 2020.

15. Gerst-Emerson K, Jayawardhana J. Loneliness as a public health issue: the impact of loneliness on health care utilization among older adults. Am J Public Health 2015;105(5):1013–9.

16. Pulselive. How official figures may hide true virus death toll. 2020. Available at: https://www.pulselive.co.ke/news/world/how-official-figures-may-hide-true-virus-death-toll/0n71pv8. Accessed June 28, 2020.

17. Holt-Lunstad J, Smith TB, Layton JB. Social relationships and mortality risk: a meta-analytic review. PLoS Med 2010;7(7):e1000316.

18. Sorkin D, Rook KS, Lu JL. Loneliness, lack of emotional support, lack of companionship, and the likelihood of having a heart condition in an elderly sample. Ann Behav Med 2002;24(4):290–8.

19. The oldest old and the 90+ Study. Available at: https://www.ncbi.nlm.nih.gov/pmc/articles/PMC3373258/. Accessed June 29, 2020.

20. What is Dementia?. Available at: https://www.nia.nih.gov/health/what-dementia-symptoms-types-and-diagnosis. Accessed June 29, 2020.

21. Suicide Risk Highest in Older Men. Available at: https://www.psychiatryadvisor.com/home/topics/suicide-and-self-harm/suicide-risk-highest-in-older-men/. Accessed June 29, 2020.

22. Isolated and struggling, many seniors are turning to suicide. Available at: https://www.npr.org/2019/07/27/745017374/isolated-and-struggling-many-seniors-are-turning-to-suicide. Accessed June 29, 2020.

23. Zhang B, Wang HE, Bai YM, et al. Inflammatory bowel disease is associated with higher dementia risk: a nationwide longitudinal study. Gut 2020;70(1):85–91.

24. Lauriola M, Mangiacotti A, D'Onofrio G, et al. Neurocognitive disorders and dehydration in older patients: clinical experience supports the hydromolecular hypothesis of dementia. Nutrients 2018;10(5):562.

25. Archibald C. Promoting hydration in patients with dementia in healthcare settings. Nurs Stand 2006;20(44):49–52.

26. Prevalence of obesity and severe obesity among adults: United States, 2017-2018. NCHS Data Brief 2020;(360):1–8. Available at: http://search.ebscohost.com/login.aspx?direct=true&AuthType=shib&db=mdc&AN=EPTOC142098114&site=eds-live. Accessed June 28, 2020.

27. Hales CM, Carroll MD, Fryar CD, et al. Prevalence of obesity and severe obesity among adults: United States, 2017-2018. NCHS Data Brief 2020;(360):1–8.

28. Sleep Foundation.org. White paper: how much sleep do adults need?. Available at: https://www.sleepfoundation.org/professionals/whitepapers-and-position-statements/white-paper-how-much-sleep-do-adults-need. Accessed June 10, 2020.

29. McCall C, Winkelman JW. The use of hypnotics to treat sleep problems in the elderly. Psychiatr Ann 2015;45(7):342–7.

30. Ancoli-Israel S, Cooke JR. Prevalence and comorbidity of insomnia and effect on functioning in elderly populations. J Am Geriatr Soc 2005;53(7 Suppl):S264–71.

31. Ohayon MM. Epidemiology of insomnia: what we know and what we still need to learn. Sleep Med Rev 2002;6(2):97–111.

32. Bloom HG, Ahmed I, Alessi CA, et al. Evidence-based recommendations for the assessment and management of sleep disorders in older persons. J Am Geriatr Soc 2009;57(5):761–89.

33. Chen W. Does more sleep time improve memory? evidence for the middle-aged and elderly. Am J Health Ed 2019;50(6):366–73.

34. Kitching D. Depression in dementia. Aust Prescr 2015;38(6):209–2011.

35. Satlin A. Sleep disorders in dementia. Psychiatr Ann 1994;24(4):186–91.

36. Culnan E, McCullough LM, Wyatt JK. Circadian rhythm sleep-wake phase disorders. Neurol Clin 2019;37(3):527–43.

37. Sletten TL, Magee M, Murray JM, et al. Efficacy of melatonin with behavioural sleep-wake scheduling for delayed sleep-wake phase disorder: a double-blind, randomised clinical trial. PLoS Med 2018;15(6):e1002587.

38. Hoyos CM, Gordon C, Terpening Z, et al. Circadian rhythm and sleep alterations in older people with lifetime depression: a case-control study. BMC Psychiatry 2020;20(1):1–9.

39. Stone KL, Xiao Q. Impact of poor sleep on physical and mental health in older women. Sleep Med Clin 2018;13(3):457–65.

40. Rubiño JA, Gamundí A, Akaarir M, et al. Bright Light Therapy and Circadian Cycles in Institutionalized Elders. Front Neurosci 2020;14:1. Available at: http://search.ebscohost.com/login.aspx?direct=true&AuthType=shib&db=edb&AN=143100880&site=eds-live. Accessed July 6, 2020.

41. Tortosa-Martínez J, Clow A, Caus-Pertegaz N, et al. Exercise increases the dynamics of diurnal cortisol secretion and executive function in people with amnestic mild cognitive impairment. J Aging Phys Act 2015;23(4):550–8.

42. Scher C, Meador L, Van Cleave JH, et al. Moving beyond pain as the fifth vital sign and patient satisfaction scores to improve pain care in the 21st Century. Pain Manag Nurs 2018;19(2):125–9.

43. By the 2019 American Geriatrics Society Beers Criteria® Update Expert Panel. American Geriatrics Society 2019 updated AGS Beers Criteria® for potentially inappropriate medication use in older adults. J Am Geriatr Soc 2019;67(4):674–94.

44. Varteresian T, Lavretsky H. Natural products and supplements for geriatric depression and cognitive disorders: an evaluation of the research. Curr Psychiatry Rep 2014;16(8):456.

45. Nair BR, Browne W, Marley J, et al. Music and dementia. Degener Neurol Neuromuscul Dis 2013;3:47–51.

46. Health Benefits of T'ai Chi. Available at: https://www.health.harvard.edu/staying-healthy/the-health-benefits-of-tai-chi. Accessed June 29, 2020.

47. Cramer H, Anheyer D, Lauche R, et al. A systematic review of yoga for major depressive disorder. J Affect Disord 2017;213:70–7.

48. Thorsteinsson G. Chronic pain: use of TENS in the elderly. Geriatrics 1987;42(12):75–82.

49. Kang KY. Effects of visual biofeedback training for fall prevention in the elderly. J Phys Ther Sci 2013;25(11):1393–5.

50. Consider Ice and Heat. Available at: https://www.webmd.com/pain-management/try-heat-or-ice. Accessed July 4, 2020.

51. Koncicki HM, Unruh M, Schell JO. Pain Management in CKD: A Guide for Nephrology Providers. Am J Kidney Dis 2017;69(3):451–60.

52. Lloyd SL, Striley CW. Marijuana Use Among Adults 50 Years or Older in the 21st Century. Gerontol Geriatr Med 2018;4. 2333721418781668.

53. Beedham W, Sbai M, Allison I, et al. Cannabinoids in the older person: a literature review. *Geriatrics* (Basel) 2020;5(1):2.
54. Available at: https://www.statista.com/statistics/588027/medical-marijuana-patients-oregon-age. Accessed July 14, 2020.
55. Ducharme J. COVID-19 is making america's loneliness epidemic even worse. 2020. Available at: https://time.com/5833681/loneliness-covid-19/. Accessed July 14, 2020.
56. Wortham JM, Lee JT, Althomsons S, et al. Characteristics of persons who died with COVID-19 — United States, February 12–May 18, 2020. MMWR Morb Mortal Wkly Rep 2020;69:923–9.
57. Lake J. A mental health pandemic: the second wave of COVID-19. Available at: https://www.psychiatrictimes.com/view/a-mental-health-pandemic-the-second-wave-of-covid-19. Accessed June 14, 2020.
58. Feuer W. Doctors worry the Coronavirus is keeping patients away from US hospitals as ER visits drop: heart attacks don't stop'. 2020. Available at: https://www.cnbc.com/2020/04/14/doctors-worry-the-coronavirus-is-keeping-patients-away-from-us-hospitals-as-er-visits-drop-heart-attacks-dont-stop.html. Accessed June 20, 2020.
59. Kaiser Health News. Nearly half of Americans delayed medical care due to pandemic 2020. Available at: https://khn.org/news/nearly-half-of-americans-delayed-medical-care-due-to-pandemic/. Accessed June 20, 2020.
60. Roberts ET, Mehrotra A. Assessment of disparities in digital access among medicare beneficiaries and implications for telemedicine. JAMA Intern Med 2020. https://doi.org/10.1001/jamainternmed.2020.2666.
61. Lam K, Lu AD, Shi Y, et al. Assessing telemedicine unreadiness among older adults in the United States during the COVID-19 pandemic. JAMA Intern Med 2020. https://doi.org/10.1001/jamainternmed.2020.2671.
62. Robinson JL, Corrada MM, Kovacs GG, et al. Non-Alzheimer's contributions to dementia and cognitive resilience in The 90+ Study. Acta Neuropathol 2018; 136(3):377–88.
63. Parkar SR. Elderly mental health: needs. Mens Sana Monogr 2015;13(1):91–9.
64. World Health Organization. Mental health of older adults. 2017. https://www.who.int/news-room/fact-sheets/detail/mental-health-of-older-adults. Accessed July 28, 2020.
65. Lêng CH, Wang JD. Daily home gardening improved survival for older people with mobility limitations: an 11-year follow-up study in Taiwan. Clin Interv Aging 2016;11:947–59.
66. The healing power of pets for seniors. Available at: https://www.agingcare.com/Articles/benefits-of-elderly-owning-pets-113294.htm. Accessed June 29, 2020.
67. More evidence that pets benefit mental health. Available at: https://www.medicalnewstoday.com/articles/325795. Accessed June 29, 2020.

Traits Versus States
Understanding Personality Disorders

Lisa Tannenbaum, PA-C[a,b], Melissa Rodzen, PA-C[c],*

KEYWORDS

- Personality disorders • Dimensional-categorical hybrid model
- Psychiatric taxonomy

KEY POINTS

- Personality disorders have onset by early adulthood and are marked by inflexible, maladaptive personality dysfunction.
- The classification of personality disorders is a topic of current research and is expected to change significantly in upcoming years.
- Terminology, vocabulary, and even categorization of personality disorders can be convoluted, vague, or redundant at times.

INTRODUCTION

It is estimated that as many as 1 in 10 people have some form of personality disorder, but many of these individuals do not seek care and remain undiagnosed.[1] Lack of treatment is caused in part by the changing and evolving landscape of psychiatric medicine. Personality disorders have been recognized for thousands of years but have been explained historically by various rationales, including imbalance of the humors, so-called moral insanity, and neurologic degeneration. The pathophysiology of personality disorder is still the subject of research. This ongoing research itself also leads to diagnostic confusion because the definition of personality disorder changes over short periods of time. In the 1920s, Kurt Schneider formally classified patients with personality disorder as those who "suffer because of their disorders and also cause society to suffer."[2] Although this definition is vague, it remains the foundational concept of personality disorder.

The Diagnostic and Statistical Manual on Mental Disorders, Fifth Edition (DSM-5), released in 2013, defines personality disorder as an "enduring pattern of inner experience and behavior that deviates markedly from the expectations of the individual's culture, is pervasive and inflexible, has an onset in adolescence or early adulthood,

a Victory Recovery Partners (VRP), Massapequa, NY, USA; b Bel Air Center for Addictions, 1202 Brighton Lane, Bel Air, MD 21014, USA; c NYU Langone Emergency Department, 150 55th Street, Brooklyn, NY 11220, USA
* Corresponding author.
E-mail address: melissa.rodzen@nyulangone.org

Physician Assist Clin 6 (2021) 467–477
https://doi.org/10.1016/j.cpha.2021.02.008
2405-7991/21/© 2021 Elsevier Inc. All rights reserved.
physicianassistant.theclinics.com

is stable over time, and leads to distress or impairment."[3] Personality disorders occur when pathologic personality traits are pervasive, are not normal characteristics of development, and are not otherwise a direct result of other physiologic influences such as substance use. Personality change caused by medical conditions may also occur, but such changes are diagnostically distinct from the 10 predominant personality disorders defined by the DSM-5 and discussed in this article.

JINGLES AND JANGLES

The process of diagnosing and treating psychiatric illnesses has formalized the definitions over the last century. Several concepts and terminologies have conflicting, congruent, or even mixed connotations compared with their historical usage. Further ambiguity has been caused by jingle fallacies and jangle fallacies, even in scholarly literature.

- Jingle fallacy: referring to different constructs using the same word[4]
  o Example: referring to both a lethargic and stuporous patient using the term lethargic
- Jangle fallacy: using multiple words to describe the same construct[4]
  o Example: referring to feelings of anxiety as anxiety, nerves, and worry

The use of standardized, updated vocabulary in professional settings is imperative to limit the confusion and misrepresentation of patients with psychiatric disease. When relevant, commonly misused terminology and concepts are clarified in this article with respect to describing and understanding personality disorders.

DIFFICULT PATIENTS

In an attempt to accommodate different viewpoints and reduce the complexity surrounding classification of personality disorder, the DSM-5 abandoned personality axis. However, it did keep the cluster categorization of personality disorder. Section III of the Personality Disorder chapter in the DSM-5 introduces proposed research topics for reconceptualization of these disorders into a dimensional model. It is possible that the cluster categorization system will be replaced in the future. However, at present, the core concepts for personality disorders remain intact.

A Marked Deviation

Personality disorder is consistently described as behavior and patterns of thinking that are not typical of an individual's culture or stage of development. This behavior may be a deviation of cognition, affectivity, interpersonal functioning, or impulse control.

Pervasive over Time and Situation

An individual with personality disorder shows inflexible, maladaptive traits beginning in early adulthood that result in functional impairment across a variety of circumstances and consistently over time; for instance, in multiple work, school, and home environments. This behavior is in contrast with impulsivity only expressed during a manic episode. Patients with personality disorder do not experience asymptomatic periods, because the symptoms of personality disorder are pervasive and constant by definition.[3]

Traits Versus States

It is generally accepted that any personality contains a spectrum of various traits and characteristics that can be considered favorable or unfavorable in any given culture or circumstance. The distinction between a personality trait and a personality disorder is an important one. Individuals who are easily angered and impulsive do not necessarily have a personality disorder, although they may show mood lability and poor impulse control. It is when these traits are rigidly present despite changes in environment or situation, causing functional impairment or distress, that they become suspicious for disorder. Although not diagnostic, the example in **Box 1** helps to illustrate the differences between typical personality traits and the inflexible, pervasive traits of personality disorder.

CLUSTER A: THE ODD OR ECCENTRIC

Cluster A disorders are described as asocial and withdrawn.[2] Disorders in this category are often diagnosed in individuals who avoid interactions with other people and frequently misinterpret events around them. Those with cluster A disorders may experience brief psychotic episodes.

Paranoid Personality Disorder

Paranoid personality disorder (PPD) describes a pervasive distrust of others. Although it is true that many people are distrusting from time to time, individuals with PPD are extreme in their distrust. They often lack any basis for their suspicions, but believe others are attempting to cause them harm or fool them in some way. This belief is not limited to a single contact and extends beyond prejudice toward entire groups. Patients with PPD are preoccupied with asking themselves why others act the way they do and looking for ways in which others are trying to deceive, demean, exploit, or otherwise negatively affect them. Patients with PPD often limit contact with others and, when they spend time with friends, they may withhold information or even lie about details for fear that any information will be used as a weapon against them. In a typical conversation, patients with PPD may perceive hidden motivations behind comments, gestures, facial expressions, or tones of voice that others understand to be benign and ordinary.

Box 1
Personality trait versus personality disorder

Personality Trait	Personality Disorder
Joe is described by his friends as a hothead. He frequently gets into fights in bars and has trouble maintaining an appropriate level of calm when he feels provoked. Even his coworkers note he is frequently agitated and comment that they are concerned about his stress levels. Joe himself acknowledges that he sometimes loses control of his anger and acts impulsively as a result. However, he finds he is able to manage his anger at home to maintain his relationship with his wife and 2 children. Although he is sometimes violent with strangers, he is never violent with his family or friends. He is actively involved in his community and is frequently rewarded in his career for above-average work performance and 15 y of dedication to the company	Joe is described by his friends as a hothead. He frequently gets into fights in bars and has trouble maintaining an appropriate level of calm when he feels provoked. His inability to control his anger has resulted in multiple arrests, divorce from his wife, and limited visitation rights with his children. He has lost several jobs because of his violence in the workplace, and storms out of interviews if he is not quickly offered a position after a few minutes of discussion. Others in the community state they are wary of Joe when he is around and even avoid bars he is known to frequent to dodge his aggressive behaviors. When interviewed, Joe simply acknowledges his actions, stating those affected by his violence "deserved what they got" for making him angry

People with PPD, along with those with other cluster A disorders, tend to avoid interactions with others and are generally not considered mood labile. However, people with PPD may quickly respond with anger and even respond aggressively to perceived attacks or slights, whether or not the transgression is validated by others. When offended, these individuals often show a propensity to be unforgiving and may use a negative event as evidence that confirms their distrust of others.

Schizoid Personality Disorder

Schizoid personality disorder describes pervasive detachment from others and a restricted range of emotional expression, often resulting in a flat affect even when the patient is directly praised or criticized (**Box 2**).[3] People with schizoid personality disorder are often described as loners. They tend to prefer solitary activities, do not seek out the company of others, and frequently lack desire for sexual intimacy or romantic relationships. However, unlike those with PPD, individuals with schizoid personality disorder are usually uninterested in the motivations, opinions, and/or actions of others. These patients typically lack the cognitive and perceptual distortions often observed in patients with schizotypal personality disorder. The absence of these distortions may be useful for differentiation.[3]

Special care should be taken to differentiate schizoid personality disorder from depressive episodes and autism spectrum disorder, especially in younger populations, because they have many overlapping features. Age of onset and progression of disease may be useful for differentiation. High-functioning autism and schizoid personality disorder overlap to a great degree; both may show restricted affect and impaired understanding or response to social cues. However, individuals with high-functioning autism often do not meet full criteria for schizoid personality disorder despite shared traits.[5]

Schizotypal Personality Disorder

Schizotypal personality disorder is described by a pattern of so-called magical thinking, cognitive or perceptual distortions, and often ideas of reference (**Box 3**). Patients frequently have oddities of speech, mannerisms, and patterns of dress; they are viewed as eccentric. Similar to those with schizoid personality disorder, schizotypal patients typically avoid close relationships with others and prefer solitude. These patients usually have few social relationships outside of first-degree relatives, and may be increasingly uncomfortable in social settings even with known people in familiar surroundings. The difference between this discomfort and social anxiety is that, in patients with schizotypal personality disorder, discomfort around others often originates from feelings of paranoia.

Box 2
Mood versus affect

Mood is how the patient reports feeling; it is subjective and internal. Affect is how the patient appears to an observer. Affect may or may not be congruent with mood.

For example, a patient feeling depressed may put on a happy face for family. This patient is showing a happy affect despite a reported depressed mood. Patients with schizoid personality disorder may have a flat or depressed affect and they usually do not report extreme variations of mood.

This point may be an important distinguishing feature when differentiating a state of depression from schizoid personality disorder.

> **Box 3**
> **Schizotypal personality disorder**
>
> **A change in the wind**
>
> In the DSM-5, schizotypal personality disorder is described as both a personality disorder and a psychotic and schizophrenia-spectrum disorder. The history of schizotypal personality disorder and other schizophrenia-spectrum disorders is convoluted, and stems from an attempt to differentiate psychotic from subpsychotic or borderline disorders in the early 1900s.
>
> In the 1970s, subpsychotic and/or borderline schizophrenia was renamed schizotypal and categorized as a personality disorder. The most recent version of DSM-5 reclassifies schizophrenia as a spectrum disorder with the inclusion of schizotypal personality disorder under this umbrella. Further research is underway to investigate boundaries between these disorders, especially in reference to the risk of psychosis.[6]

- Ideas of reference
  - Interpreting particular meaning or personal significance to external events. For example, believing a thunderstorm is a result of one's anger.
- Delusions of reference
  - Ideas of reference held with strong conviction despite evidence contrary to the belief. Delusions of reference may indicate psychosis.

CLUSTER B: THE DRAMATIC, EMOTIONAL, OR ERRATIC

Cluster B disorders are often described as explosive disorders with features of mood lability, impulsivity, and self-serving behaviors.[2] Although cluster A disorders are considered disorders of social withdrawal and limited expression, cluster B disorders are disorders of intense emotional instability.

Antisocial Personality Disorder

Antisocial personality disorder is described as a pattern of pervasive disregard for the rights, feelings, or desires of others.[3] Colloquially, people with antisocial personality disorder are often described as psychopaths or sociopaths. Individuals with antisocial personality disorder fail to abide by literal or conventional laws of society and repeatedly find themselves in arguments and/or physical altercations. Patients may be violent, intentionally aggressive, manipulative, or deceitful, and often show an inability to responsibly fulfill occupational, financial, familial, or other social obligations (**Box 4**). Although individuals with antisocial personality disorder act without regard for the rights, feelings, or desires of others or may act intentionally to cause harm, they also lack remorse or guilt and often justify their actions with superficial or overly simplistic reasoning.[3]

This disorder is considered so highly stigmatized that there are restrictions to diagnosis because of the assumed severity of disease and implications of diagnosis (**Box 5**). Unlike other personality disorders, antisocial personality disorder cannot be diagnosed before age 18 years, and, even then, symptoms must have been present since age 15 years.[3]

In pediatric patients, characteristics suggestive of developing antisocial personality disorder (patterns of aggression toward people or animals, destruction of property, deceitfulness, or serious rule violations) may instead be diagnosed as conduct disorder.[3]

Box 4
Antisocial

Antisocial: more than a little shy

The term antisocial should be used in reference to antisocial personality disorder as described earlier. Antisocial is not a synonym for introversion, which is better described in a medical setting using the term asocial. Asocial indicates a lack of social behaviors or interactions and a general withdrawal from others.[4]

Borderline Personality Disorder

Borderline personality disorder is defined as a pattern of instability in interpersonal relationships, self-image, and affects, and marked impulsivity.[3] Patients with borderline personality disorder may be described as unpredictable, with sudden changes in behavior or affect. They are often sensitive to changes in circumstance or environment, especially if the change is perceived as a threat of abandonment. Individuals with borderline personality disorder may respond with rage when notified by family members that their flight to visit was canceled because of a storm. Although the circumstances are definitively out of either party's control, the family members may be accused of not caring about the patient or not trying hard enough to visit, which is perceived as willful abandonment.

Patients with borderline personality disorder always show patterns of relational instability, affect, and self-image. They may rapidly oscillate between idealization and vilification of caregivers, children, friends, or colleagues.

Small changes may ignite extreme emotional response in patients with borderline personality disorder. Episodes of dysphoria, anger, irritability, anxiety, or panic may last only minutes or hours. Colloquially, these changes are often described by others as mood swings (**Box 6**). Periods of intense emotion and impulsivity may be accompanied by self-mutilation, suicide attempts, or threats of self-harm. These behaviors are sometimes used as manipulation tactics to make others prove love or show that they are there for the patient, to relieve fears of abandonment. However, up to 10% of patients with borderline personality disorder die by suicide. Thus, such threats should always be treated appropriately.[7]

Individuals with borderline personality disorder may or may not retain insight. They may see themselves as all good or all bad, similarly to how they view others, or they may feel empty with only a vague sense of their own identity (**Box 7**). Some people with borderline personality disorder may even transiently show dissociative symptoms.[3]

Box 5
Sociopathy and psychopathy

The terms sociopath and psychopath both have multiple imprecise and sometimes overlapping definitions. Historically, they were used to describe characteristics of antisocial personality disorder. The concept of psychopathy is still used mainly as a description of antisocial traits, particularly in personality tests. Older editions of the DSM referenced "sociopathic personality disturbances," but both psychopathy and sociopathy as concepts have been absorbed by the distinct diagnosis of antisocial personality disorder. Although the DSM-5 does acknowledge the existence of the terms sociopath, psychopath, and dissocial personality disorder, it makes no distinction among them. The use of these phrases is thus ill-advised.

> **Box 6**
> **Bipolar disorder versus borderline personality disorder**
>
> Although the term mood swings is often used to describe bipolar disease, this is misleading. The mood patterns of bipolar disease most frequently occur as episodes of mania, hypomania, or depression lasting several days or weeks at a time. Although mood lability is common, fluctuations do not typically confuse the predominant mood state of the episode. In between episodes (usually no more than 2–3/y) individuals with bipolar disease experience asymptomatic periods lasting weeks, months, or even years.
>
> However, individuals with borderline personality disorder may have shifting predominant moods over the course of hours or even minutes without a single predominant mood state. They rarely experience extended asymptomatic periods. By definition, the instability and impulsivity associated with borderline personality disorder are pervasive and not a result of other mood disorders (though other disorders may coexist).

Narcissistic Personality Disorder

Narcissistic personality disorder is a pattern of grandiosity, need for admiration, and lack of empathy.[3] Like many personality disorders, narcissistic personality disorder is frequently misunderstood even by medical professionals. Narcissistic traits are common; however, as with other personality disorders, these traits must be pervasive, inflexible, and must cause dysfunction or distress to meet criteria for disorder. These patients possess an exaggerated sense of their abilities and seek admiration and validation from others. They often believe they are better than other people and may think they are misunderstood by anyone who they do not perceive to be equally high status.

Individuals with narcissistic personality disorder take advantage of other people and maintain unreasonable expectations of others. They are unwilling or unable to acknowledge the needs, wants, or emotions of others, while simultaneously expecting their own needs and wants to be addressed by others.

Histrionic Personality Disorder

Histrionic personality disorder presents as a pattern of showing excessive emotion and attention-seeking behaviors.[3] These patients are often social and enjoy being the center of attention; they go out of their way to maintain the attention of others. Individuals with histrionic personality disorder often dress flamboyantly to further draw attention to themselves and often spend significant time and resources on their appearance.

In clinical settings, they may capture attention by describing dramatic compilations of symptoms, which frequently change in an attempt to be engaging. They may be overly flattering, open with personal details, or even be sexually forward. Histrionic patients frequently verbalize strong opinions despite superficial understanding or knowledge of details with which to form the foundations of the opinion. Similarly, individuals

> **Box 7**
> **Splitting**
>
> Splitting is a characteristic of patients with borderline personality disorder in which the individual perceives others as entirely good or bad.
>
> The term is often misused colloquially in medicine to describe a patient attempting to generate conflict between caregivers.[8]

with histrionic personality disorder may form opinions of others with limited information and interpret relationships to be more intimate than they actually are. For example, when describing a new friend, someone with histrionic disorder may say "She's like the sister I never had. I can't imagine life without her," despite having met only 1 week prior.

However, theatrical displays of emotion expressed in histrionic disorder are not always positive. Individuals may argue or sob loudly in public or frequently shift moods depending on responses elicited from surroundings. Individuals often go to great lengths in order to maintain the attention of others.

CLUSTER C: THE ANXIOUS OR FEARFUL

Cluster C personality disorders are described as depressive, avoidant, or anxious.[2]

Avoidant Personality Disorder

Avoidant personality disorder is described as a pattern of social inhibition, feelings of inadequacy, and hypersensitivity to negative evaluation.[3] These patients often avoid interpersonal contact, not because of paranoia or anxiety but because of fears of rejection or criticism. Individuals with avoidant personality disorder are very risk averse in social situations and often show inhibition or avoid social interactions completely, unless they are certain they will be liked. Despite appearing withdrawn and quiet, people with avoidant personality disorders do have interest in social relationships but are inhibited by fears of shame or ridicule (**Box 8**). They have pervasively low self-esteem and feelings of inadequacy and intensely fear criticism, embarrassment, and rejection.

Dependent Personality Disorder

Dependent personality disorder is a pervasive and excessive need to be taken care of that leads to submissive and clinging behavior and fears of separation.[3] Individuals with dependent personality disorder often struggle with daily decisions. They require reassurance and advice, and go to great lengths in order to receive support from others. Individuals with dependent personality disorder struggle with responsibility and are reluctant to initiate projects because they depend on others to take leadership roles. These patients are often fearful of being alone or being forced to care for themselves because of pervasive feelings of inadequacy and incompetence.

Obsessive-Compulsive Personality Disorder

Obsessive-compulsive personality disorder (OCPD) is a pervasive pattern of preoccupation with orderliness, perfectionism, and control.[3] This preoccupation with details is so extensive that it overshadows the activity being organized. Someone with OCPD may find completing projects difficult because of exorbitant amounts of time spent trying to reach overly strict personal standards (**Box 9**). These patients may hoard both worthless objects as well as those worth more (ie, money). This hoarding

---

Box 8
Avoidant versus anxious

Avoidant personality disorder and social anxiety disorder can be remarkably similar to each other and nearly impossible to distinguish.

This overlap is so extensive that they are sometimes considered to be the same condition. It is common for patients to carry both diagnoses.[3]

Box 9
Obsessions versus compulsions

Obsessions	Compulsions
Recurrent and persistent thoughts, urges, or images that are experienced as intrusive or unwanted[3] Obsessions are anxiety provoking[4]	Repetitive behaviors or mental acts that an individual feels driven to perform in response to an obsession or according to rules that must be applied rigidly[3] Compulsions relieve anxiety caused by obsessions[4]

OCD, unlike OCPD, involves the presence of obsessions and compulsions[3]

Individuals with OCD are distressed by obsessions, but those with OCPD think their rigidity serves a purpose

Abbreviation: OCD, obsessive-compulsive disorder.

---

behavior is often centered on a need for preparedness and control rather than greed. A focus on productivity and perfection is so pervasive that patients may not think they have time for leisure and may view it as a waste of time that could be spent working. Similarly, play or leisure activities are likely to be structured and organized into sets of tasks.

Individuals with OCPD are rigid and uncompromising in their beliefs and rule systems. When working with others, they prefer detailed instructions to use as rules to which they strictly adhere. They expect others to follow their own set of rules and to meet their standards, even when unrealistic, and often struggle with the idea of tasks having multiple paths to completion. They are often so inflexible they prefer not to delegate tasks and instead absorb more work in order to ensure it is done right.[3]

One More Thing

The DSM-5 does not include previous disorders such as depressive, haltlose, and passive-aggressive personality disorder. It does include the miscellaneous category of other specified personality disorder and unspecified personality disorder, which may be used for diagnoses no longer included or those that do not meet the diagnostic criteria described earlier. Similarly, there are other traits, characteristics, and conditions that may influence personality without being personality disorders (**Box 10**).

TREATMENT

The lifelong nature of personality disorder and the notoriously limited effects of treatment have been a great source of frustration for clinicians for hundreds of years. Over time, personality disorders have earned reputations of being untreatable, which often leads to lack of an attempt to intervene.[9]

Traditional wisdom teaches that patients with personality disorders almost always show impaired insight, but recent research has challenged this observation

---

Box 10
Multiple personality disorder

Some may note the absence of multiple personality disorder in this article. This disorder is omitted because it is not a personality disorder at all. In 1994, the DSM-4 renamed this disorder dissociative identity disorder, which, even now, remains a controversial diagnosis.[8]

> **Box 11**
> **Insight**
>
> ## A lack of insight?
>
> The term insight is used to describe an individual's understanding of self. This term may relate to many interactions between an individual and the environment, but is most often used to describe a spectrum of an individual's awareness of behavior, emotions, or illness and how they influence an individual's interactions with the world.[10] Insight is essentially a modernization of Freud's concepts of egosyntonic and egodystonic instincts. Individuals with egosyntonic qualities do not think their behavior is incompatible with their self-image or goals. Individuals with egodystonic qualities act in ways that conflict with their self-image and goals. Those with a personality disorder who lack insight may be described as egosyntonic, suggesting they are oblivious to the destructive nature or even presence of their disorder. Egodystonic individuals recognize the traits causing dysfunction and seek to change the behavior. Such individuals are modernly be described as having insight to their condition.

(**Box 11**). Although this does not serve any diagnostic relevance, the presence or lack of insight bears significant relevance to managing personality disorder. Patients with a lack of insight often do not seek care, do not agree with diagnoses, and do not comply with follow-up or treatment recommendations. Patients with critical impairments of insight frequently do not acknowledge their illness and are unaware of how their actions contribute to negative life events. It is important to recognize the patient's level of insight, because it may explain the patient's view to the clinician and, perhaps, reduce clinician frustration.

SUMMARY

The concept of personality is universally accepted, but distinguishing personality traits from personality disorder can be difficult. This difficulty is further complicated by ambiguous, subjective, and frequently overlapping descriptions of disease, some of which are nearly impossible to objectively differentiate. This problem is especially detrimental when considering the highly stigmatized nature of some personality disorders.[11]

The DSM-5 contains proposed methods for updating to a dimensional model rather than the current categorical model in DSM-4. In the DSM-5 dimensional model, 6 of 10 personality disorders are retained, namely antisocial, avoidant, borderline, narcissistic, OCPD, and schizotypal. These disorders are to be characterized more specifically to personality function and pathologic traits rather than descriptions.[12]

The proposed International Classification of Disease (ICD)-11 system differs from the DSM-5 section III proposals in that it suggests abolishing type-specific categories of personality disorder. Instead, the ICD-11 proposition includes 1 diagnosis of personality disorder that represents a continuum with various dimensions of traits. This proposition maintains the essential definition of personality disorder while eliminating the overlap and ambiguities of the current categorical system. This classification system instead has practitioners assess personality disorder and describe individual disease rather than fitting patients into categories that are often ill-fitting and highly stigmatized.[2]

Overall, the future taxonomy and diagnostic criteria for personality disorder is an area of active debate and study. Further research is needed to understand, manage, and, if possible, prevent personality disorder. A vital step to accomplish this is the standardization of terminology and a consensus of disease definition. This step is long overdue.

CLINICS CARE POINTS

- As many as 1 in 10 people have some form of personality disorder, but many of these individuals do not seek care and remain undiagnosed.

- Imprecise terminology has led to great difficulty in describing, diagnosing and treating personality disorders throughout the history of psychiatric medicine. Accurate definitions are essential.

- A transient personality trait should be considered a personality disorder only when it is rigidly present despite changes in environment or situation, causing functional impairment or distress.

DISCLOSURE

M. Rodzen, no disclosures; L. Tannenbaum, no disclosures.

REFERENCES

1. Lenzenweger MF. Epidemiology of personality disorders. Psychiatr Clin North Am 2008;31(3):395-vi.
2. Newton-Howes G, Clark LA, Chanen A. Personality disorder across the life course. Lancet 2015;385(9969):664–734.
3. Diagnostic and statistical manual of mental disorders, fifth edition (DSM-5). American Psychiatric Association; 2013.
4. Lilienfeld SO, Sauvigné KC, Lynn SJ, et al. Fifty psychological and psychiatric terms to avoid: a list of inaccurate, misleading, misused, ambiguous, and logically confused words and phrases. Front Psychol 2015;6. https://doi.org/10.3389/fpsyg.2015.01100.
5. Yam WH, Simms LJ. Comparing criterion- and trait-based personality disorder diagnoses in DSM-5. J Abnorm Psychol 2014;123(4):802–8.
6. Lilienfeld SO, Pydych AL, Lynn SJ, et al. 50 Differences That Make A Difference: A Compendium of Frequently Confused Term Pairs in Psychology. Front Educ 2017;2:37.
7. Sleep CE, Lamkin J, Lynam DR, et al. Personality disorder traits: testing insight regarding presence of traits, impairment, and desire for change. Personal Disord 2019;10(2):123–31.
8. Marková IS, Berrios GE. The meaning of insight in clinical psychiatry. Br J Psychiatry 1992;160:850–60 [published correction appears in Br J Psychiatry 1992;161:428].
9. Schultze-Lutter F, Nenadic I, Grant P. Psychosis and schizophrenia-spectrum personality disorders require early detection on different symptom dimensions. Front Psychiatry 2019;10:476.
10. Cook ML, Zhang Y, Constantino JN. On the continuity between autistic and schizoid personality disorder trait burden. J Nerv Ment Dis 2020;208(2):94–100.
11. Paris J. Suicidality in borderline personality disorder. Medicina (Kaunas) 2019;55(6):223.
12. Tyrer P, Reed GM, Crawford MJ. Classification, assessment, prevalence, and effect of personality disorder. Lancet 2015;385(9969):717–26.

Nervous and Scared

Understanding Anxiety and Trauma/Stressor-related Disorders and Obsessive-Compulsive Disorders

Phyllis R. Peterson, PA-C, MPAS, CAQpsy[a,b,c,*],
Rodney Ho, PhD, MPH, PA-C, Psychiatry-CAQ[d]

KEYWORDS

• Anxiety disorders, Obsessive-compulsive Disorders, Interventions

INTRODUCTION

Anxiety can be normal and often is described as a brief or time-limited reaction to unknown, internal, vague, or conflictual thoughts.[1] Normal anxiety may improve alertness and performance in high-demand situations (ie, fight or flight). If persistent and/or severe, however, anxiety slows attention, performance of tasks, psychosocial function, and cognition. The *Diagnostic and Statistical Manual of Mental Health Disorders* (Fifth Edition) (*DSM-5*) reports that anxiety disorders are the most prevalent psychiatric condition.[2] Studies vary, with prevalence rates at 4.8% to 10% annually, with a 33% lifetime occurrence rate.[1,3,4]

Pathophysiology is unclear but believed to include genetic predisposition, childhood adversity, recent stress, and the interaction of plasticity markers.[1] There is a 30% inheritability risk.[2] The roles of the serotoninergic systems and neurotrophic signaling have been associated with anxiety and are the topic of research.[4] Anxiety has a worldwide incidence of 1 in 5 people. This translates to a global percentage of 3.8%, contrasted with a 3.4% worldwide depression rate and a 0.3% schizophrenia rate.[5,6] There is a large economic and humanistic burden that increases with illness severity.[7] This burden is estimated to be $42 billion for the US economy ($82 billion in 2020 dollars).[8] Approximately 10%, or $256, per anxious worker was attributed to low productivity and absenteeism, with 30% as psychiatric costs.[8] Chisholm and colleagues[9] estimate that if spending on anxiety and depression were increased from 2016 to 2030, there could be a savings in years of healthy life, which translates to a $300 billion economic impact.

[a] NP/PA Post Graduate Psychiatry Program, Texas Tech University Health Sciences Center, Lubbock, TX, USA (retired); [b] Psychiatric PA Services, Leander, TX, USA; [c] Connell & Associates, Killeen, TX, USA; [d] University of West Florida, 2614 Brad Clemmons Drive, JBSA-Lackland 78236
* Corresponding author. 2321 Broken Wagon Drive, Leander, TX 78641.
E-mail address: psychpa@hotmail.com

Physician Assist Clin 6 (2021) 479–493
https://doi.org/10.1016/j.cpha.2021.03.002
2405-7991/21/© 2021 Elsevier Inc. All rights reserved.
physicianassistant.theclinics.com

Aristotle described anxiety in the third century BC, and it has figured in medical commentaries across numerous cultures. Freud later coined the term, anxiety neurosis, and his description has been the basis of the *Diagnostic and Statistical Manual of Mental Health Disorders.*[10] In the most recent version, *DSM-5*, obsessive-compulsive disorders (OCDs) and posttraumatic stress disorder (PTSD) were removed from the anxiety classification and given a separate classification.[2] Separation anxiety and selective mutism (SM), disorders found more frequently in children, were moved into the anxiety classification, allowing this diagnosis to be applied to adults.[11]

Anxiety disorders can cause dysfunction in 1 or more areas of a person's life. This dysfunctional response to worry can manifest as somatic or peripheral symptoms, neuropsychic symptoms, and/or behavioral symptoms.[2,3] **Table 1** is the replication of index card the author (P.R. Peterson) used this on an index card for many years.

Differential diagnosis of anxiety includes psychotic disorders (including schizophrenia), mood disorders, adjustment disorder, and avoidant personality. Medical causes that can present with anxiety include cardiac disease (ie, angina, heart failure, arrhythmias, and myocardial infarction), thyrotoxicosis, pheochromocytoma, carcinoid, embolism, pain, hypoxia, hypoglycemia, and/or Meniere disease. Medications causing anxiety include antipsychotics, aminophylline, sympathomimetic agents, and psychostimulants as well as withdrawal from thyroid medications/benzodiazepines/hypnotics.[2,12,13]

Evaluation of anxiety disorders should rule out medical and substance causes, including adverse reactions and drug-drug interactions. There is high comorbidity between anxiety disorder and the depressive disorders, OCD, avoidant personality disorder, and/or substance use disorders (SUDs).[12] Differentiating among the anxiety disorders can be challenging, but using a table may help (**Table 2**).

Anxiety disorders are under-recognized in primary care practices and thus undertreated. During the pandemic of 2020, there were growing concerns of increasing episodes of anxiety disorders, and clinicians were urged to be mindful of likely increased incidence of mental health disorders.[14] Patients presenting with a suspected anxiety disorder require a thorough review of systems, medical, psychiatric, family, medication, and psychosocial history. These patients often present with fear and worry regarding the evaluation itself, and establishment of a therapeutic alliance can take time. Utilization of measurement-based treatment and following evidence-based guidelines can help increase the possibility of treatment to remission versus just

Table 1 Manifestations of anxiety systems[23]		
Peripheral	**Neuropsychic**	**Behavioral**
Light-headed/dizzy	Worry	Avoiding/social withdrawal
Restless	Fear	Undue time/effort spent on worry
Tachypnea/palpitations	Time distortions	Irritability
Sweating	Physical distortions	No risk taking/trying new things
Muscle tightness	Slow cognition	Not taking advantage of opportunities: Social, occupational, or relational
Tingling extremities	Inattention	Inability to complete tasks
Butterflies in the gut		May appear oppositional
Pupillary mydriasis		Inability to fulfill social roles
Syncope		High substance use rates

Table 2
Differentiation of anxiety disorders[2,12,13]

	Generalized Anxiety Disorder	Panic Disorder	Social Anxiety Disorder	Specific Phobia	Agoraphobia	Separation Anxiety
Average age of onset (y)	20+	24	13	7	20	Preschool, young child
Clinical course	Chronic with fluctuation, declines after age 50	Chronic Waxes and wanes	Starts slowly Chronic 1 of 8 patients develops SUD	Varies	Varies, waxes and wanes	Generally resolves, some risk of anxiety disorders
Epidemiology	2F:1 M	M = F		>F	>F	3%–4% child 1%–2% adults
Family history	+ + + + + +					
Clinical	Worry re: common everyday things, bad outcomes, avoidance, seeks reassurance	Sudden attacks, avoidance	Fear and worry re: situation with negative judgment, avoidance	Fears specific action, place, activity, or thing	Fear of being in 2 of 5 situations 6 mo, cognitive and physical avoidance	Anxiety, detachment from significant figures × 4 wk (child) × 6 mo (adult)
Initial management	CBT, SSRI, SNRI, buspirone, benzo, β-blockers	CBT, SSRI, SNRI, benzo, β-blockers	CBT, SSRI, SNRI, buspirone, benzo, β-blockers	CBT, rarely benzo	CBT, SSRI, SNRI, Benzo, β-blockers	Individual, family treatment, CBT SSRI
US lifetime prevalence[a]	6.2%	5.2%	13%	13.8%	2.6%	

Abbreviations: benzo, benzodiazepine; F, female; M, male.
[a] Per National Comorbidity Survey, data prior to *DSM-5* removing OCD and PTSD.

improvement. Remission allows patients to become and stay fully functional able to reach their full potential.[12–14] Scales used to screen for and follow course of treatment include the following[15–19]:

- General Anxiety Disorder-7
- Screen for Child Anxiety Related Disorders, for ages 8 to 16
- Hamilton Anxiety Scale, Patient Health Questionnaire 9
- Depression Anxiety Stress Scale (Psychology Foundation of Australia)[19]*

* Always remember that screening scales may point in a direction but psychiatric history and clinical findings lead to a diagnosis.

Treatment strategies and specific pharmacologic and psychotherapy guidelines are similar for anxiety disorders and should be utilized in a stepwise manner. In particular, cognitive-behavior therapy (CBT) as a stand-alone treatment or in combination with medication is efficacious.[1,12,14] In pediatrics, anxiety disorders are common, with one-third of the population having at least 1 disorder. It is recommended that these disorders be evaluated and treated early to avoid the consequences of underachievement, learning problems, relationship issues, or the higher risk of development of more severe anxiety disorders, SUDs, and suicidality.[20]

GENERALIZED ANXIETY DISORDER

Criteria for generalized anxiety disorder (GAD) include excessive anxiety and worry regarding hard to control events, must be present more days than not, and causing dysfunction for greater than or equal to 6 months. Three of the following must be present:

- Restlessness
- Insomnia
- Fatigue
- Poor concentration
- Irritability
- Muscle tension

The worry of GAD is pervasive, excessive, persistent, and distressing to the patient. GAD also interferes with normal function and interpersonal relationships in contrast to normal, manageable worry.[2]

Onset usually is in the early 20s and is chronic but can wax and wane over time. Worsening from "always anxious" to dysfunctional may occur with life changes (college or death of life partner), illness, or with major depressive episode. Increased risk factors include family history (33% higher), age (prior to 30), female gender (2-times higher), and African American ethnicity.[2] Women often have more psychiatric comorbidities (ie, depression) whereas men have more SUDs. Symptoms have a cultural presentation; some cultures accept physical symptoms more readily and this may lead to more peripheral complaints versus neuropsychic.[2,3]

Treatment of anxiety includes biologics (medication and neuromodulation) along with therapy (CBT, psychoanalysis, supportive therapy, and individual or group therapy).[21–23] Alternative modalities, such as nutritional and lifestyle changes (mindfulness, meditation, exercise, and yoga), have less robust evidence of efficacy.[22,23] They generally are encouraged, however, to enhance overall health and wellness and may help individuals and do no harm. Not all patients need medication if their anxiety is mild and function is not unduly affected. If medication is used, however, treatment may take some weeks to be effective.[24] Sleep is important and initially should be treated with sleep hygiene techniques, CBT, a sleep study (if needed), and, as a last resort, medication.[22,24] CBT is the cornerstone of nonbiologic treatment. CBT can be provider-based (therapist or primary care provider) or directed with workbooks and online resources if a therapist is not accessible. Patients should be encouraged to explore and identify techniques that help them and incorporate these techniques into their daily lives. In more severe or complicated cases, patients should be referred for in-person psychotherapy.

The most frequent medications used in the treatment of GAD include selective serotonin uptake inhibitors (SSRIs), selective serotonin-norepinephrine uptake inhibitors (SNRIs), tricyclic antidepressants (TCAs), benzodiazepines, and buspirone (**Box 1**). After selecting an initial antidepressant, it should be taken to the optimal dose and an adequate time trial assure. If the medication is ineffective or not tolerated, a switch to another approved medication should be considered. When a partial response is seen, the cause (ie, nonadherence, pharmacokinetic variables, or placebo effect) should be considered and either medications switched or present treatment augmented.[12–14,24]

Other medications, used off label, include antihistamines, atypical antipsychotics, and pregabalin. For GAD, there are 3 SSRIs and 2 SNRIs with efficacy demonstrated in randomized controlled trials (RCTs) and FDA approved: escitalopram, paroxetine, sertraline, duloxetine, and venlafaxine. Use of off-label medication should be discussed with the patient and side effects need to be monitored, especially QT interval prolongation and hepatic function.

Once remission is achieved, treatment should continue for 6 months to 18 months because GAD tends to be chronic.[24] Some patients may be able to reduce medication dosage or eliminate one from an augmented regimen if CBT and/or lifestyle modifications (sleep hygiene or lifestyle changes) have been helpful. Patients should be encouraged to seek early follow-up if symptoms return or worsen.

Transcranial magnetic stimulation (TMS) has been studied recently for anxiety. Although it is not approved for anxiety, TMS has been found efficacious in some studies for anxiety and trauma disorders. One type of TMS is approved for OCD.[26]

Box 1
Generalized anxiety disorder medication[12,13,23,25]

Start with an approved SSRI; if not effective or not tolerated:
1. Switch to second standard medication
2. Switch to either another class or within class:
   a. A second SSRI
   b. From an SSRI to an SNRI
   c. From an SNRI to an SSRI
   d. From an SSRI to a TCA
   e. From an SNRI to a TCA
   f. To buspirone
3. Use a nonstandard medication:
   a. Hydroxyzine
   b. Benzodiazepine (fast-acting positive effect on somatic and autonomic symptoms)
   c. Pregabalin
4. Augment present treatment:
   a. Hydroxyzine: no trials as augmentation but some support moderate effectiveness alone
   b. Propranolol: no trials
   c. Buspirone: STAR*D (the Sequenced Treatment Alternatives to Relieve Depression trial) results do not support
   d. Pregabalin: 1 augmentation trial with small effect
   e. Benzodiazepine: no augmentation trials, effective alone
   f. Atypical antipsychotics: only if psychotic due to high risk of metabolic effects

Psychedelics for depression and anxiety have been used since the 1960s. Clinical trials administering psilocybin have demonstrated possible resetting of brain networks that may be efficacious in psychiatric disorders.[27,28] Additionally, studies in virtual reality for anxiety and panic disorders (PDs) are hopeful. Medications under research include some promising results from modulators of glutamate neurotransmitters (ketamine and riluzole xenon), a neurosteroid (Aloradine), and several medications that may accelerate fear extinction and thus speed up exposure therapy (MDMA [3,4-methylenedioxymethamphetamine], L-DOPA [levodopa or l-3,4-dihydroxyphenylalanine] , cannabinoids, and D-cycloserine).[29] Treatment of last resort is neuromodulation surgery.[30,31] Surgery includes ablation (destroying an area of the brain) or selective stimulation (implanting a device to modulate neural networks).[29]

PANIC DISORDER

PD presents with a powerful surge of fear and discomfort. Episodes reach an apex in minutes (5–20), generally arise suddenly, and during an episode exhibit at least 4 of the following symptoms:

- Fear of losing control
- Fear of dying
- Palpitations
- Sweating
- Trembling
- Shortness of breath
- Choking–throat tightening
- Dizziness
- Chills or heat sensitivity
- Nausea or GI distress
- Paresthesia
- Derealization[2]

Attacks are followed by a month or more of persistent worry that another attack will occur and thus the patient adopts changes in behavior aimed at avoiding an episode. Symptoms cannot be medical in origin nor related to a different mental disorder (ie, trauma, obsessions, or phobias) and cannot appear only in response to social situations.[2] Although some patients report attacks lasting hours, this likely represents ongoing worry about further attacks.[2]

First episodes often prompt emergency department visits. Patients then are referred to the specialty based on the physical symptoms, which may lead to extensive unnecessary evaluations or even procedures. A good history and review of symptoms, including psychiatric, physical examination, and basic laboratory tests, are needed to rule out medical causes (ie, hyperthyroidism, hypoglycemia, supraventricular tachycardia, and pheochromocytoma). The incidence of PD is estimated at 5% for women and 2% for men.[6] The onset is typically in the 20s, rarely after age 30.

The course of PD generally is chronic but treatment with medications and psychological therapy usually is effective. Causes of PD appear to be genetic and biological. There is a 20% rate of the disorder among first-degree relatives.[6] Although targeted genes are not identified, twin studies indicate a higher rate of PD among identical versus fraternal twins. Biologically, PD is mediated by locus coeruleus abnormality, carbon dioxide hypersensitivity, abnormal lactate metabolism, increased catecholamines, and γ-aminobutyric acid abnormalities.[2,4]

RCTs support initial treatment with either psychosocial or pharmacologic interventions. Psychosocial interventions include CBT as monotherapy (if no mood disorder) and often is the treatment of choice. Panic-focused psychodynamic psychotherapy has some evidence as well. Pharmacologic treatment includes SSRIs, SNRIs, TCAs (if no mood disorder), or a benzodiazepine.[12,23] There is no compelling evidence of 1 medication superiority. The choice of initial therapy should include patient preference, risk/benefit, cost, availability, past or first-degree relative effectiveness, and dosing. Evaluation of effectiveness can be complicated as antidepressants can take several weeks to be effective and to evaluate their effect on attacks. Even benzodiazepines, which generally show some benefit in the first week, can take several weeks to fully stop attacks. It generally is recommended to wait a minimum of 6 weeks, with 2 weeks at full dose, before changing medications.[32] CBT benefits often do not accrue until 12 sessions, and patients may have become adept at avoiding triggers. They may be reluctant to give that up to test effect and challenge dysfunctions; this fear lessens symptom reporting and skews evaluation. When treatment is ineffective or only partially effective, the clinician should revisit the diagnosis, looking for complicating factors, such as SUDs or adherence.[1,12]

When switching medications after the first trial, the standard is similar to the guidelines in GAD. Switches can be cross-titrated in most instances. For a partial response, after 2 trials of an SSRI or SNRI, add CBT, TCA, or a benzodiazepine. Buspirone is not effective in PD. If CBT was the initial treatment, adding a medication may be helpful and this decision should be made in consultation with the therapist.[21–23]

Following exhaustion of standard treatment options, mirtazapine and gabapentin have shown modest effectiveness, and pindolol augmentation has some preliminary support (although no other β-blockers). Antipsychotics are not recommended due to limited evidence of effectiveness and side effects. Monoamine oxidase inhibitors (MAOIs) are regarded as effective for PD but are limited by their safety profile and patients taking MAOIs need to adhere to a low-tyramine diet and a 2-week washout period. The need for more complicated regimens or secondary or tertiary medication regimens usually is handled by specialists.[12,14,32] No studies have compared the various behavioral therapies in PD. Eye movement desensitizing and reprocessing therapy (EMDR) have some data in PD and trauma; however, there was poor functional recovery at 3-month follow-up, so it is not routinely recommended.[32]

POSTTRAUMATIC STRESS DISORDER

PTSD was introduced in the *DSM* (Third Edition), in 1980, in response to experiences from many patients, notably Vietnam War veterans.[33] PTSD has been studied extensively with war veterans and is synonymous with other wartime diagnoses, such as shell shock, stress syndrome, battle fatigue, and traumatic war neurosis.[34]

PTSD is a chronic and potential debilitating psychiatric disorder that develops after exposure to a traumatic event that must entail a threatened or actual death, serious injury, or sexual violence.[2] The lifetime prevalence of PTSD is estimated to be 6.4% in the general population and higher in women (8.6%) compared with men (4.1%). Rates of PTSD are higher among veterans and other occupations that carry an increased risk of traumatic exposure, including police officers, firefighters, and emergency personnel.[2] The probability of developing PTSD varies across cultural groups after exposure to a traumatic event. US Latinos, Native Americans, and African Americans have higher rates compared with US non-Latino Whites; Asian Americans have the lowest rates of PTSD.

According to the *DSM-5*, there are 7 diagnostic criteria (criteria A–H) required to meet a diagnosis of PTSD. Each criterion (A–H) has a set number of symptoms that must be present to fulfill that criterion.[2] Criterion A requires exposure to 1 or more traumatic event (ie, threatened or actual death, serious injury, or sexual violence). The event can be experienced directly or witnessed; learned about from an actual or threatened traumatic event experienced by a friend or relative; or repeated exposure to details of a traumatic event (eg, military members repeatedly exposed to combat-related deaths).

Criterion B includes intrusive symptoms beginning after the traumatic event. One of the following symptoms must be present to meet this diagnostic criterion:

- Repeated and unwanted intrusive memories of the traumatic event
- Distress dreams about or related to the event
- Flashbacks (experiences or acts if the traumatic event is happening again)
- Strong physical reactions to internal or external stimuli related to the traumatic event

Avoidance symptoms are common in PTSD and are reflected in criterion C of the *DSM-5*. Criterion C is met if there is 1 avoidance symptom (ie, individuals suffering from PTSD avoid places, object, or situations) or a marked effort to avoid conversations, places, or individuals that remind the patient of the trauma or bring up memories of the traumatic event.

Criterion D is negative beliefs of self and the world manifested by the individual.[2] The individual is unable to recall an important part of the traumatic event, has recurring feelings self-blame and guilt, and may feel disconnect or removed from others. Criterion D is meet when 2 symptoms of negative alterations in beliefs and mood occur or are worsened following the experience of the traumatic event.[2]

Criterion E requires 2 symptoms of alterations in reactivity and arousal to be present or worsen after a traumatic event. The common symptoms of reactivity and arousal are irritability or aggression, difficulty concentrating, difficulty sleeping, and hypervigilance. Criterion F refers to the duration of the symptoms in criteria B, C, D, and, E and must be at least 1 month or more. Lastly, criterion G states the symptoms cause considerable distress and interfere with important parts of life (ie, occupational, social, and personal).[2]

PTSD has been diagnosed in children as young as 6. There are separate criteria for those children younger than 6, a population susceptible to traumatic events, such as child or sexual abuse. Disturbing memories of the traumatic event(s) and hypervigilance typically dominate the initial phase of PTSD. The chronic phase of PTSD is dominated by symptoms of negative beliefs of oneself, the world, and the presence of negative emotions. A diagnosis of acute stress disorder is similar to the diagnostic criteria of PTSD; however, acute stress disorder symptoms are present from 3 days to 1 month following a traumatic event whereas PTSD requires the duration to be a minimum of 1 month.

A majority of individuals who experience a traumatic event do not develop PTSD and exhibit normal acute reactions, such as intrusive thoughts, irritability, and problems with sleep and memory.[35] Studies have shown that the prevalence of PTSD increases proportionally as the exposure to traumatic events increases. PTSD is more likely to occur following exposure to severe forms of trauma, such as rape or military combat. Risk of development of PTSD is associated with a family history of psychiatric disorders, female gender, lower socioeconomic status, lower education/intelligence, childhood trauma, prior mental disorders (ie, depressive disorder and PD), and racial and ethnic minority groups.[2]

Assessment of Posttraumatic Stress Disorder

A through assessment is essential for an accurate diagnosis and effective treatment. The *DSM-5* PTSD criteria should guide the assessment and ongoing evaluation of symptom severity during treatment. Initial PTSD screening tools recommended by the Veterans Affairs (VA) are the Primary Care PTSD Screen (PC-PTSD) and the PTSD Checklist for *DSM-5* (PCL-5).[36] Diagnosis should be made based on a clinical interview or a structured diagnostic interview, such as the Clinician-Administered PTSD Scale for *DSM-5* or PTSD Symptom Scale—Interview for *DSM-5*.[36] PTSD is associated with other comorbid mental disorders, such as major depressive disorder, and leads to a reduction of quality of life, physical health, and functional impairment. These outcomes should be assessed during a comprehensive diagnostic evaluation.

Treatment of Posttraumatic Stress Disorder

Studies have shown that trauma-focused psychotherapy is more effective in reducing core PTSD symptoms than pharmacotherapies.[36] The VA PTSD Clinical Practice Guideline Work Group recommends trauma-focused psychotherapies, such as prolonged exposure therapy, cognitive processing therapy, EMDR, specific CBT for PTSD, brief electric psychotherapy, oral narrative exposure therapy, and/or written narrative exposure.[36] When trauma-focused psychotherapy is not available, non–trauma-focused psychotherapy, such as CBT, is recommended. Sertraline, paroxetine, and fluoxetine are specific SSRIs that have shown to be effective monotherapy for the treatment of PTSD.[36] Venlafaxine, an SNRI, also is an effective PTSD monotherapy treatment.

SOCIAL ANXIETY DISORDER

SAD has an annual prevalence higher in the United States than anywhere else in the world (7% vs 0.5%–2%, respectively).[2,3] SAD is characterized by excessive, persistent, and distressing fear and anxiety caused by social interactions. Patients fear they will present as anxious or be thought of as crazy, weak, or worse. This fear of being judged negatively, rejected, or offending to others leads to avoidance. Although patients report fear/anxiety is worse in some situations, almost all social situations provoke some degree of anxiety. In pediatrics, to be diagnosed with SAD, the symptoms must occur in situations with both peers and adults. SAD criteria require 6 months of symptom duration.[2]

Onset of social anxiety occurs generally between ages 8 and 13. It can be insidious or follow a particularly stressful event. It rarely develops in adulthood but can be a reaction following significant life changes. There likely is some genetic predisposition because there is a 2-times to 6-times greater risk in first-degree relatives.[2] Differential diagnoses include other anxiety disorders, mood disorders, OCD, avoidant personality, and eating disorders. SAD also can coexist with other mental health disorders. Clinically these individuals often are anxious in the clinic/interview, with restricted verbal responses.[2,12,14]

Treatment is similar to that for anxiety and PD. Fluoxetine, sertraline, paroxetine, and long-acting venlafaxine all are approved for SAD. TCAs are not effective. Other SSRIs and SNRIs are likely effective but off-label. MAOIs are effective but should be reserved, if possible, for resistant cases due to medication side-effect profile. Benzodiazepines are effective in SAD but should be used cautiously. Propranolol is efficacious for performance anxiety and can be dosed on either as-needed or used off-label as daily dosing. CBT can be helpful in addressing thought patterns and reactions; generally, exposure, desensitization and flooding are the techniques of choice.[12,14,21,23]

SPECIFIC PHOBIAS

Specific phobias affect 12% of the population with onset between ages 18 and 59.[6] The essential criteria include fear and anxiety and occur nearly every time the person is near the object or in the situation. The object generally is something that potentially could harm, but the fear and anxiety usually are out of proportion to the danger. The anxiety persists and can cause significant psychosocial distress and dysfunction.[2] Most patients fear more than 1 object or situation and the disorder tends to run in families.[18] The differential and comorbidities are the same as SAD; however, treatment should focus on CBT. Medications generally are not indicated, although benzodiazepines can be used carefully for specific situations.

AGORAPHOBIA

Prior to *DSM-5*, agoraphobia was not an individual diagnosis but a qualifier or specifier of PD. It is uncommon, occurs slightly more in women than men, and begins in adolescence. The lifetime prevalence of agoraphobia is thought to be approximately 1.3%; however, as a new *DSM* category, there are limited data.[2,3,6] Risks are stratified into temperamental (eg, neuroticism, sensitivity to anxiety, and anxiety disorders), environmental (childhood trauma, reduced warmth, or overprotectiveness), and genetic and physiologic predisposition.[37]

DSM-5 criteria include having excessive, pervasive fear, or anticipatory anxiety about 2 or more of 5 situations:

- Using transportation
- Open spaces
- Closed spaces
- Crowded spaces
- Being away from home alone

Criteria also include avoidance brought on by the situation.[2] Symptoms are persistent (≥6 months). It is rare, but in the worst cases, patients become totally homebound. The fear is characterized by anxiety about ability to escape the situation in case of a panic attack or panic-like episode. Differential diagnosis includes PD, SAD, MDD, PTSD, separation anxiety, or acute stress.[2,12,14] In mild cases, CBT (exposure therapy) may be sufficient; in more severe cases, treatment can include SSRIs, SNRIs, TCAs, or benzodiazepines.[12,37]

OBSESSIVE-COMPULSIVE DISORDER

OCD is a chronic psychiatric disorder that causes marked distress and impairment in all aspects of life. Those afflicted with OCD experience intrusive and recurrent troubling thoughts using repetitive behaviors or mental acts to reduce anxiety.[38] OCD has a lifetime prevalence of 2.3% and the mean age of onset of 19.5 years.[2] OCD affects more women compared with men; however, men have an earlier age onset.

OCD is characterized by 2 distinct diagnostic indicators: obsessions and compulsions. Obsessions are manifested by persistent unwanted and unpleasant thoughts or urges to perform a behavior. Compulsions are rituals, repetitive behaviors, or mental acts that an individual feels the need to perform due to an obsession. These are based on rules that must be rigidly followed. Individuals afflicted with OCD suffer from both obsessions and compulsions. Some common examples of obsessions are thinking about contamination, symmetry, or forbidden thoughts (ie, sexual, religious, or those of fear of harm to oneself or others).[2] Compulsions are the behaviors that respond to the obsession, such as cleaning (washing hands), ordering, counting items, or continuously checking on something.

OCD was removed from the anxiety chapter of *DSM-5* and placed in a separate chapter. The new chapter is named, "Obsessive-Compulsive and Related Disorders," which includes hoarding disorder, body dysmorphic disorder trichotillomania (hair-pulling disorder), and excoriation (skin-picking) disorder. These mental health disorders have common diagnostic features and validators.[2]

OCD is a potentially debilitating psychiatric disorder with a delayed diagnosis. Once OCD is diagnosed, patients and their loved ones should be educated regarding the diagnosis and treatment. The baseline and monitoring of OCD symptoms during treatment can be done by using standardized rating scales or by the patient report of the time spent on obsessions and compulsions and the level of distress. An example of a common standardized scale is the Yale-Brown Obsessive-Compulsive Scale—Second Edition, which is a reliable tool for assessing OCD symptom severity.[38] SSRIs are considered the first-line psychopharmacologic treatment of OCD. Paroxetine, fluoxetine, sertraline, and fluvoxamine are approved for the treatment of OCD; however, citalopram and escitalopram commonly are used off-label.[38] To ensure adequate treatment, higher doses of SSRIs usually are needed and the dose should be titrated over 4 weeks to 6 weeks. Psychopharmacologic treatment should continue for a minimum of 2 years, although, in some cases, medication may be needed indefinitely. This often is due to patient preference and/or severity of OCD symptoms and distress. The gold standard of psychological treatment of OCD is CBT, exposure, and response prevention.[38] If an adequate trial of an SSRI (6 weeks) or psychological therapy does not result in a satisfactory response, the combined treatment should be attempted.

SEPARATION ANXIETY

Separation anxiety is a fear or anxiety about separation from persons or places to which a person has strong attachments. This fear is not developmentally appropriate and out of proportion to the situation. There is fear of bad occurrences when away from attachment figures, manifesting itself as a refusal or reluctance to go out, sleep away from home, or go to sleep. The patient may have nightmares and refuse to be alone. In pediatrics, the criteria require symptoms for 4 weeks whereas in adults, persistent symptoms must occur for greater than or equal to 6 months with significant disruption of function.[2]

Separation anxiety occurs most often in preschool children and can continue into the preteen years. Concurrent anxiety disorders may develop but often these are a response to trauma, stressful situations, changes in family structure, moves, or displacement. Comorbidities include any of the anxiety disorders, oppositional defiant disorder, conduct disorder, PTSD, bereavement, depression, psychosis, and personality disorders.[2,13]

Treatment includes a combination of behavior and medication. Therapy type is dependent on the age of patient; younger children may need play therapy, positive reinforcement, and graded exposure. Therapy must include family and parental guidance.[13] Older children and adults generally benefit from CBT and medication because they often have comorbid psychiatric conditions.

SELECTIVE MUTISM

Refusal to speak in specific social situations while being able to speak in others (school vs home) is an essential criterion for SM. Symptoms must be consistent and occur for greater than or equal to 1 month. Dysfunction in education and social function also occur. SM cannot be due to lack of knowledge/comfort with the spoken language nor disorders of communication (ie, stuttering). SM cannot be diagnosed in autism, schizophrenia, or other psychotic disorders.[2] Controversy has occurred with the removal of SM from childhood disorders and the move to anxiety disorders. This move occurred because the anxiety component of SM may lead to increased diagnosis in adults. SM is considered a preliminary diagnosis with a need for a deeper dive into comorbidities and coexisting developmental disorders. Often, SM is the initial presentation, leading to the discovery of neurocognitive deficits of auditory processing. These deficits determine type and course of effective treatment.[11]

The condition is rare, with an incidence of 0.3% to 1% nationally (variable due to survey setting). It is seen mainly in young children and infrequently in adolescence and adults. Comorbidities and differential diagnoses include separation, social anxiety, specific phobia, and oppositional behavior. Treatment is challenging and may include SSRIs, behavior therapy with positive reinforcement, contingency management, assertiveness training, and parental counseling.

ANXIETY DISORDERS CONCLUSION AND CLINICAL POINTS

- General medical evaluation is an essential part of good psychiatric care.
- Evaluation and intervention for general medical problems help with psychiatric treatment.
- Assess for trauma and chronic stressors.
- Assess for nonsuicidal (self-harm) and suicidal thinking, behavior, or attempts.
- Complete medication history and drug-drug interaction evaluation should be undertaken to limit adverse reactions.
- The most common comorbidities of anxiety are attention-deficit/hyperactivity disorder, depression, and SUDs.
- Evaluate and treat concurrently.
- Ask about bullying or intimidation (children and adults).
- Adjustment disorder often is due to a specific event or situation and time limited.
- Bipolar disorder can present as anxiety; have the patient define "anxiety."
- Autism spectrum disorder often is comorbid with anxiety and deserves treatment to eliminate worsening of core symptoms.
- Developmental disorder patients may only be able to express anxiety symptoms in behaviors.
- Some patients self-medicate then present with anxiety related to withdrawal or craving; consider SUD as the diagnosis.
- Self-care (proper nutrition and exercise) is important.
- Initially, use Food and Drug Administration (FDA)-approved medications for the various anxiety disorders.
- Benzodiazepine use should be limited to weeks or months and carefully monitored; their quick onset of action and improvement of physical symptoms are advantageous but they have a high abuse potential.
- Base treatment recommendations on symptom severity and level of distress/dysfunction.
- Mild GAD, SAD, social phobia, and panic disorder may respond to behavior techniques but most will need medication.
- Buspirone is not effective in PD.
- Caffeine should be limited in anxiety disorders.
- Avoidance of anxiety-provoking activities and situations may be reinforced by family and teachers; however, this leads to more severe disorders. Therefore, it is important to educate patients and provide therapy.
- There is some evidence that therapy can mitigate recurrence. Some patients who did not have CBT as part of initial treatment may benefit from it on stabilization.

- Anxiety disorders are associated with suicidality even in the absence of depression and patients should be evaluated regularly.
- Use validated scales for evaluation and monitoring.
- When 2 or more anxiety conditions are present, identification of the specific disorders is important in medication choice and in psychotherapy.
- Do mental status evaluations every visit.
- Treat to remission, not only improvement.
- Withdrawal of medications (especially benzodiazepines) should be done slowly and carefully while observing for a recurrence of symptoms or decline of function.
- Pharmacogenomics testing is not standard practice but can be used in some situations, such as treatment resistance.[31]

DISCLOSURE

P.R. Peterson: nothing to disclose. R. Ho: the views and written materials expressed in this publication do not necessarily represent the views of US Air Force, Department of Defense, and the US Government.

REFERENCES

1. Thibaut F. Anxiety disorders: a review of current literature. Dialogues Clin Neurosci 2017;19(2):87–8.
2. American Psychiatric Association-APA. Diagnostic and statistical manual of mental disorders (DSM-V). 5th edition. Washington, DC: Author; 2013.
3. Bandelow B, Michaelis S. Epidemiology of anxiety disorders in the 21st century. Dialogues Clin Neurosci 2015;17(3):327–35.
4. Bandelow B, Baldwin D, Abelli M, et al. Biological markers for anxiety disorders, OCD and PTSD: A consensus statement. Part II: Neurochemistry, neurophysiology and neurocognition. World J Biol Psychiatry 2017;18(3):162–214.
5. World Health Organization. Depression and other common mental disorders: global health estimates. Geneva 2017. Available at: https://www.who.int/publications/i/item/depression-global-health-estimates. Accessed August 24, 2020.
6. Hannah Ritchie and Max Roser (2018) - "Mental Health". Published online at OurWorldInData.org. Available at: https://ourworldindata.org/mental-health. Accessed August 24, 2020.
7. Toghanian S, Dibonaventura M, Järbrink K, et al. Economic and humanistic burden of illness in generalized anxiety disorder: an analysis of patient survey data in Europe. Clinicoecon Outcomes Res 2014;6:151–63.
8. Greenberg PE, Sisitsky T, Kessler RC, et al. The economic burden of anxiety disorders in the 1990s. J Clin Psychiatry 1999;60(7):427–35.
9. Chisholm D, Sweeny K, Sheehan P, et al. Scaling-up treatment of depression and anxiety: a global return on investment analysis. Lancet Psychiatry 2016;3(5):415–24.
10. Crocq MA. A history of anxiety: from Hippocrates to DSM. Dialogues Clin Neurosci 2015;17(3):319–25.
11. Holka-Pokorska J, Piróg-Balcerzak A, Jarema M. The controversy around the diagnosis of selective mutism - a critical analysis of three cases in the light of modern research and diagnostic criteria. Kontrowersje wokół diagnozy mutyzmu wybiórczego – krytyczna analiza trzech przypadków w świetle współczesnych badań oraz kryteriów diagnostycznych. Psychiatr Pol 2018;52(2):323–43.

12. Black D, Andreasen N. Introductory textbook of psychiatry. 6th edition. Washington, DC: American Psychiatric Publishing; 2014.

13. Amray AN, Munir K, Jahan N, et al. Psychopharmacology of pediatric anxiety disorders: a narrative review. Cureus 2019;11(8):e5487.

14. Mangolini VI, Andrade LH, Lotufo-Neto F, et al. Treatment of anxiety disorders in clinical practice: a critical overview of recent systematic evidence. Clinics (Sao Paulo) 2019;74:e1316.

15. Available at: https://www.crossroadscounselingcenters.com/pdf/Generalized%20Anxiety%20Disorder.pdf. Accessed August 28, 2020.

16. Available at: https://www.pediatricbipolar.pitt.edu/sites/default/files/SCAAREDAdultVersion_1.19.18.pdf. Accessed August 28, 2020.

17. Available at: https://dcf.psychiatry.ufl.edu/files/2011/05/HAMILTON-ANXIETY.pdf. Accessed August 28, 2020.

18. Available at: https://www.med.umich.edu/1info/FHP/practiceguides/depress/phq-9.pdf. Accessed August 28, 2020.

19. Available at: http://www2.psy.unsw.edu.au/groups/dass/order.htm

20. Ayers JW, Leas EC, Johnson DC, et al. Internet searches for acute anxiety during the early stages of the COVID-19 Pandemic. JAMA Intern Med 2020. https://doi.org/10.1001/jamainternmed.2020.3305.

21. Andrews G, Bell C, Boyce P, et al. Royal Australian and New Zealand College of Psychiatrists clinic practice guidelines for the treatment of manic disorder, social anxiety disorder and generalized anxiety disorder. Aust N Z J Psychiatry 2018;52(12):1109–72.

22. Abejuela HR, Osser DN. The psychopharmacology algorithm project at the harvard south shore program: an algorithm for generalized anxiety disorder. Harv Rev Psychiatry 2016;24(4):243–56. https://doi.org/10.1097/HRP.0000000000000098.

23. Osser D. Psychopharmocology Institute. GAD Pharmacotherapy: Augmenting vs Switching in partial responders. Available at: https://www.youtube.com/watch?v=E0KVnGewOzQ. Accessed September 3, 2020.

24. Puzantian T, Carlat D. The medication Fact Book for psychiatric practice. 5th edition. Newberryport: Carlat Publishing; 2020.

25. Available at: https://psychiatryonline.org/pb/assets/raw/sitewide/practice_guidelines/guidelines/panicdisorder.pdf. Accessed September 3, 2020.

26. Rodrigues PA, Zaninotto AL, Neville IS, et al. Transcranial magnetic stimulation for the treatment of anxiety disorder. Neuropsychiatr Dis Treat 2019;15:2743–61.

27. Muttoni S, Ardissino M, John C. Classical psychedelics for the treatment of depression and anxiety: A systematic review. J Affect Disord 2019;258:11–24.

28. Nichols DE, Johnson MW, Nichols CD. Psychedelics as medicines: an emerging new paradigm. Clin Pharmacol Ther 2017;101(2):209–19.

29. Sartori SB, Singewald N. Novel pharmacological targets in drug development for the treatment of anxiety and anxiety-related disorders. Pharmacol Ther 2019;204:107402.

30. Fogwe DT, Spurling BC, Mesfin FB. Neuromodulation Surgery for Psychiatric Disorders. In: StatPearls. Treasure Island (FL): StatPearls Publishing; 2020.

31. Available at: https://www.mcpap.com/pdf/AnxPearls.12.05.18.pdf. Accessed September 20, 2020.

32. Goddard AW. Morbid Anxiety: Identification and Treatment. Focus (Am Psychiatr Publ) 2017;15(2):136–43.

33. Psychiatric A. Diagnostic and statistical manual of mental disorders. 3rd edition. Washington, DC: American Psychiatric Publishing; 1980.

34. Jones JA. From nostalgia to post-traumatic stress disorder: A mass society theory of psychological reactions to combat. Int Student J 2013;05(2):1–3.
35. Lancaster CL, Teeters JB, Gros DF, et al. Posttraumatic stress disorder: overview of evidence-based assessment and treatment. J Clin Med 2016;5(11):105.
36. The Management of Posttraumatic Stress Disorder Work Group. VA/DoD Clinical Practice Guideline for the Management of Posttraumatic Stress Disorder and Acute Stress Disorder. 2017. Available at: https://www.healthquality.va.gov/guidelines/MH/ptsd/VADoDPTSDCPGFinal012418.pdf. Accessed September 20, 2020.
37. Balaram K, Marwaha R. Agoraphobia. Stat Pearls Publishing; 2020.
38. Fenske JN, Petersen K. Obsessive-Compulsive Disorder: Diagnosis and Management. Am Fam Physician 2015;92(10):896–903.

Is It Real: Understanding Psychosis

Robert Sobule, MS, PA-C, CAQ-Psychiatry

KEYWORDS

- Psychosis • Schizophrenia • Auditory hallucinations • Visual hallucinations
- Delusions

KEY POINTS

- Psychosis is a syndrome occurring when one's mind loses touch with reality.
- Hallucination can occur across all senses.
- Psychotic symptoms can occur in nonpsychiatric illnesses.
- Delusions are fixed and difficult to treat.
- Psychosis can increase risk of suicidality.

INTRODUCTION

Psychosis, what exactly does it mean? Psychosis in itself is not a disease but more of a syndrome or sequelae from other disease states or substances.[1] Psychosis is a condition where one's mind loses touch with reality. It can be composed of a variety of symptoms, most commonly hallucinations, delusions, and disorganized behavior/thoughts. Often, when someone presents with psychotic symptoms, schizophrenia comes to mind. Although psychosis is a staple in the diagnosis of schizophrenia, psychotic symptoms also can occur in a variety of mental illnesses and other nonpsychiatric conditions. Examples of psychiatric conditions that can present with psychotic symptoms include mood disorders, major depressive disorder (MDD), bipolar affective disorder, and posttraumatic stress disorder (PTSD). Even severe anxiety can lead one to develop psychotic symptoms. There are several disorders identified in the Diagnostic and Statistical Manual of Mental Disorders, 5th Edition (DSM-5), which encompass psychosis, such as schizophreniform disorder, schizoaffective disorder, and substance-induced psychotic disorders. A variety of substances, both illicit and prescribed, can cause psychosis. Delirium is a common cause of psychosis, whereas other issues (eg, migraines, seizures, prion diseases, and/or insomnia) can also lead to psychotic symptoms.

There are several hypotheses on the development of psychotic symptoms. Studies have focused on patients with schizophrenia to better understand psychosis. The

---

Department of Psychiatry, University of Missouri School of Medicine, 1 Hospital Drive, Columbia, MO 65212, USA
E-mail address: Sobuler@health.missouri.edu

Physician Assist Clin 6 (2021) 495–503
https://doi.org/10.1016/j.cpha.2021.02.009
2405-7991/21/© 2021 Elsevier Inc. All rights reserved.

dopamine theory figures largely in the presumed causes of psychosis. Psychotic symptoms of schizophrenia (hallucinations and delusions) have been linked to dopamine D_2 receptor hyperactivity in the brain. Patients with schizophrenia also can have negative symptoms, social withdrawal, blunted affect, poverty of speech, and/or anhedonia, which are tied to hypoactivity of dopamine D_1 receptors. Other explanations of psychosis include dysregulation of neurochemicals, glutamate, GABA, acetylcholine, and serotonin, which are normally found in the brain.[2] Although research on psychotic symptoms has led to multiple theories behind the development of psychosis, the goal of this article was to provide a better understanding on the etiology of various *"classic"* symptoms of psychosis: hallucinations and delusions.

HALLUCINATIONS

Hallucinations are perceptions of a sense without any observable stimulus. Hallucinations can occur in any of the 5 senses: auditory, visual, olfactory, gustatory, and tactile. Hallucinations are not limited to a single sense; rather they often can affect multiple senses at once or be intermittent. Auditory and visual hallucinations are more commonly experienced than olfactory, gustatory, or tactile hallucinations. In schizophrenia, 75% of diagnosed individuals report experiencing auditory hallucinations and 16% to 72% report experiencing visual hallucinations.[3,4] Hallucinations are not limited to schizophrenia diagnoses and can occur in a variety of both psychiatric and nonpsychiatric illnesses.

AUDITORY HALLUCINATIONS

Auditory hallucinations are sounds in the absence of any auditory stimuli. They can range from nonsensical or nonverbal sounds to whispers, commands, or even yelling.[3] Auditory hallucinations can be described as occurring either from within one's head or externally. Nonverbal hallucinations are often described as tapping, animal sounds, musical notes, or songs. Historically, external hallucinations have been suggestive of more severe mental illness; however, more recently, it has been suggested that there is no concrete association between severity of illness and perceived location (inside vs outside of one's head) of hallucinations.[5] In psychiatric illness, the most commonly reported auditory hallucinations are voices. These hallucinations can have different voices/accents/inflections than those of the patient and can be either a singular voice or multiple different voices. The voices may be recognized as from a familiar person or the patient may not recognize the voice at all; voices of imaginary/fictional characters have been reported as well.

Auditory hallucinations are a hallmark symptom of schizophrenia, but they also occur in up to 50% of patients with bipolar disorder, 40% with PTSD, and 10% with MDD (**Table 1**).[3,6] Up to 40% of patients without a diagnosed psychiatric disorder report experiencing auditory hallucinations. Auditory hallucinations thought to be indicative of a psychiatric etiology tend to occur more frequently and with higher complexity while evoking more emotional response from the patient. Of note, co-occurring delusions increase the likelihood of an underlying psychiatric disorder.

Where do the voices originate? Referring back to the dopamine theory suggests that overactive dopaminergic activity in the striatum is responsible for the development of auditory hallucinations. Using PET scans, Abi-Dargham and colleagues[7] traced dopamine activity, finding increased dopaminergic activity in the brains of patients with psychotic disorders reporting auditory hallucinations. In a similar study of nonpsychotic individuals reporting auditory hallucinations, there was no increased dopaminergic activity found in the striatum, suggesting antipsychotic medications

Table 1
Psychiatric disorders associated with auditory hallucinations[6]

Thought disorders	Schizophrenia, Schizoaffective disorder, Brief psychotic episode, Schizophreniform disorder
Mood/Affective disorders	Major depressive disorder, bipolar disorder
Anxiety disorders	Generalized anxiety disorder, panic disorder
Obsessive compulsive and related disorders	Obsessive compulsive disorder, body dysmorphic disorder
Trauma and stressor-related disorders	Acute stress disorder, posttraumatic stress disorder
Personality disorders	Schizotypal personality disorder, borderline personality disorder

(dopamine antagonists) may likely not be beneficial for this population.[7] Dopamine is not the only neurotransmitter associated with auditory hallucinations. Other studies have found associations between elevated levels of glutamate, particularly in the temporal and frontal regions of the brain in patients with schizophrenia reporting frequent auditory hallucinations.[7] There are multiple hypotheses regarding structural abnormalities of various brain regions to explain the presence of auditory hallucinations. One commonly suggested theory is that auditory hallucinations stem from dysfunction in the inner speech and language processing centers of the brain. These abnormalities result in impairment of distinguishing between one's own thoughts and those of external alien origin.[3] Neuroimaging studies in patients with auditory hallucinations have shown activity in the regions of the brain associated with language comprehension, such as Broca's area and the primary auditory complex. Another theory attributes auditory hallucinations to memory deficiencies. In one study, researchers were able to identify abnormalities in the memory-forming regions of the brain in patients with schizophrenia.[3] Other studies of patients reporting auditory hallucinations have associated deficits in the prefrontal cortex and dysfunction in communication between frontal and posterior areas of the brain.[3]

There is also evidence of nonstructural or physiologic factors that have contributed to the development of auditory hallucinations. Auditory hallucinations have been reported in socially isolated individuals. It has been hypothesized that isolation or loneliness can lead to "*compensatory hypersensitivity*" of one's perceptions; one may experience auditory hallucinations to meet social needs.[7] Trauma and anxiety can lead to one developing auditory hallucinations as well.

Auditory hallucinations also can occur in a variety of nonpsychiatric illnesses: temporal lobe epilepsy, delirium, dementia, brain lesions, strokes, seizures, infections, iatrogenic (medications), and/or drug intoxication (**Table 2**).[6] For patients experiencing

Table 2
Nonpsychiatric disorders associated with auditory hallucinations[6]

Neurocognitive disorders	Alzheimer, Parkinson
Neurologic disorders	Seizure disorders, migraines, encephalitis
Neurologic insults	Stroke, tumors/lesions, traumatic brain injury, hearing loss
Sleep disorders	Narcolepsy, various parasomnias
Medications	Steroids, dopaminergic medications

auditory hallucinations without an identifiable psychiatric diagnosis, the auditory hallucinations oftentimes may be more positive in their messages and occur with less frequency and intrusiveness.

VISUAL HALLUCINATIONS

Like auditory hallucinations, visual hallucinations also can occur in a variety of different illnesses, both psychiatric and nonpsychiatric (**Table 3**).[6] Visual hallucinations have been reported in up to 72% of patients diagnosed with either schizophrenia or schizoaffective disorder.[3] Although auditory hallucinations are the most commonly reported hallucination associated with schizophrenia, there is a high incidence of visual hallucinations. Visual hallucinations in schizophrenia are often quite vivid and can manifest in a variety of forms: family members, friends, religious figures, or even animals. Visual hallucinations are associated with more severe illness in patients with schizophrenia. Hallucinations in psychiatric disorders do not typically involve distortions in size, are seen in color, and remain relatively intact regardless if the eyes are open or closed. Substance-induced visual hallucinations distort size as well change when eyes or open or closed.[8] In a depressed patient, visual hallucinations can be indicative of severity in MDD. These hallucinations can occur in both manic and depressive episodes of bipolar disorder. In mood disorders, visual hallucinations can be described as either mood-congruent or mood-incongruent. In trauma-related disorders such as PTSD, the patient may report vivid flashbacks or visualize intrusive elements related to the trauma. Visual hallucinations have been reported in personality disorders, particularly borderline personality disorder. For all their frequency, with regard to psychiatric illnesses, visual hallucinations are still poorly understood. Unlike auditory hallucinations, visual hallucinations have not been studied nearly as much in depth in relation to psychiatric illness; concentrated in exploring visual hallucinations with nonpsychiatric etiology.

From an anatomic and physiologic perspective, there are many theories of how visual hallucinations are manifested. A range of nonpsychiatric pathologies and complications can lead to one experiencing visual hallucinations (**Table 4**).[6] Simple visual hallucinations are thought to be caused by irritations of the primary visual cortex, as it is known that lesions of the visual system may cause visual hallucinations.[4]

Visual hallucinations are a hallmark symptom of delirium. Alcohol and other intoxicants can prime visual hallucinations, particularly in the context of delirium tremens (DTs) and stimulant intoxication. Patients going through DTs or stimulant intoxication often report seeing insects crawling on their skin or in their immediate environment. Many other intoxicants are known to cause visual hallucinations: ecstasy, lysergic acid diethylamide (LSD), phencyclidine (PCP), and/or psilocybin (magic mushrooms). Medications such as atropine, steroids, or dopamine agonists also can lead to iatrogenic visual hallucinations.

Table 3
Psychiatric disorders associated with visual hallucinations[6]

Thought disorders	Schizophrenia, Schizoaffective disorder, Brief psychotic episode, Schizophreniform disorder
Mood/Affective disorders	Major depressive disorder, bipolar disorder
Trauma and stressor-related disorders	Acute stress disorder, posttraumatic stress disorder
Personality disorders	Borderline personality disorder

Table 4 Visual hallucinations and possible etiology[4]	
Characteristics of Visual Hallucinations	Possible Etiology
Simple patterns, spots, shapes, lines with associated headache	Migraine, seizure disorder, brain tumor
Changing of size (large or small)	Seizure disorder, CJD
Hypnagogic	Insomnia, narcolepsy
Frightening/disturbing	Psychotic disorders, delirium, drug intoxication
Patient has good insight	Migraines, CBS

Abbreviations: CBS, Charles Bonnet syndrome; CJD, Creutzfeldt-Jakob Disease.

Teeple and colleagues explored the etiology of visual hallucinations in a variety of illnesses. They found visual hallucinations were reported in 20% of patients with Lewy body dementia (LBD).[4] These included objects moving rather than complex scenarios including people. Patients with LBD had more insight into their hallucinations than those with a primary thought disorder. There exists a strong correlation between Lewy bodies developing in the amygdala and parahippocampus and patients describing well-formed visual hallucinations.[4] Visual hallucinations can occur in other dementias, Parkinson or Alzheimer disease, although an 83% positive predictive value occurs with patients reporting visual hallucinations and a diagnosis of LBD.[3]

Charles Bonnet syndrome (CBS) occurs when visual hallucinations develop after vision loss.[4] Visual hallucinations in CBS are detailed and quite vivid to the patient. Patients with this disorder often develop fair insight into their hallucinations; they recognize what they see is unlikely to be real, as they know they are visually impaired. The visual hallucinations in CBS are attributed to a cortical release phenomenon that leads to disinhibition and sudden neuronal firings in the cortices.[4]

Almost one-third of patients with migraines report visual aura. These visions are typically described as flickering or lines that move from one periphery to another leaving trails across their field of vision and lasting less than 30 minutes.[4]

Visual hallucinations can occur in a variety of seizure disorders. Patients with seizure disorders will often describe hallucinations that are simple, brightly colored, and/or consist of shapes. Bizarre or dreamlike visual hallucinations that occur when falling asleep (hypnagogic) or on awakening are often associated with sleeping disorders such as narcolepsy and/or insomnia. Visual hallucinations have been reported in prion diseases such as Creutzfeldt-Jakob disease (CJD). Visual distortions, such as metamorphopsia and micropsia, that may occur in CJD lead to distressing visual hallucinations.[4]

TACTILE HALLUCINATIONS

Tactile hallucinations can present in a multitude of different sensations. They can be perceived as pain, stretching sensations, heaviness, touching, or changes in temperature or proprioception. Tactile hallucinations reported in schizophrenia are typically bizarre. Delusional parasitosis is a condition in which patients believe they are experiencing a parasiticlike infestation despite no evidence; they may complain of painful stimuli from "bites" or feel the perceived parasite infesting and moving around on or within them. Epigastric hallucinations have been reported in affective disorders such as bipolar and MDD. There have been limited studies investigating tactile hallucinations and their causes. A functional MRI scan of a patient with schizophrenia reporting being "*touched by spirits*" found activation of corresponding somatosensory and posterior parietal cortices when he was experiencing the tactile hallucination.[9] Another study incorporating electroencephalogram scans with reported tactile hallucinations revealed similar findings.[7]

Tactile hallucinations also occur in nonpsychiatric illnesses. One of the more common tactile hallucinations reported is "*phantom limb syndrome*" with pain affecting up to 85% of postoperative patients.[9] In phantom limb hallucinations, following amputation of a limb, patients report tactile sensations and at times debilitating pain occurring in the amputated limb. Tactile hallucinations reported in seizure disorders are often described as vague sensations that rise from epigastrium up to the throat.[10] These hallucinations also have been reported in cases of multiple sclerosis.[10]

OLFACTORY AND GUSTATORY HALLUCINATIONS

Olfactory and gustatory hallucinations are much less common than the other forms of hallucinations. Both are often associated with psychoactive substance abuse such as LSD and PCP.[11] Patients with PTSD may report olfactory hallucinations stemming from the original trauma, such as the smell of cologne from an abuser. Abnormal signaling from olfactory neurons or trigeminal nerve signals can cause olfactory hallucinations.[12] Gustatory hallucinations can occur when one loses acuity of taste sensation from allergies, illness, or traumatic brain injury.[13] Patients with seizure disorders have also reported gustatory hallucinations.

DELUSIONS

Apart from hallucinations, another common symptom in psychosis is delusions. Delusions are fixed beliefs/ideas that are clearly false and indicative of abnormal thought content.[14] Delusions can be so pervasive that no matter what evidence can be provided or rational discussion to be had to disprove one's delusions, the delusions remain. Although many may have similar types of delusions (paranoia, a commonly observed delusion), specific delusions are typically not shared; although there is some evidence for shared delusions, this is referred to as folie à deux.[6] One must consider a person's culture, religion, and level of intelligence when evaluating for delusions. Delusions can be difficult to differentiate from overvalued ideas. With delusions, there is absolutely no level of doubt; the patient's belief is 100% real to them. Overvalued ideas are also false beliefs but are less intense in that one may have some level of doubt to the validity of their thought.[6] Delusions may present in a wide variety of psychiatric disorders including schizophrenia, schizoaffective disorder, delusional disorder, or affective disorders. Delusions also can occur in substance-induced disorders; paranoid delusions are seen frequently in methamphetamine-induced psychosis. Neurocognitive disorders such as delirium or various dementias can present with delusions. The DSM-5 has multiple classifications of delusions: persecutory, referential, grandiose, erotomanic, nihilistic, and somatic. Delusions also can be classified as bizarre (clearly implausible and not understandable to peers of the same culture and do not derive from ordinary life experiences) or nonbizarre (situations that could be plausible).[14] **Table 5** further explains the different classifications of delusions.[6]

Multiple theories have been postulated on the etiology of delusions. The clinical efficacy of antipsychotic medications in treating acutely psychotic patients with both delusions and hallucinations argues for a dopamine link. Positive response to antipsychotics suggests dopaminergic hyperactivity, particularly in the mesolimbic

Table 5 Types of delusions[6]		
Type of Delusion	**Description**	**Example**
Persecutory	Belief that one is going to be harmed or is being harassed; most commonly reported delusions	"The Masons are bugging my home"
Referential	Certain gestures, comments, cues are directed at oneself; for example, ideas of reference	"The protests are my fault"
Grandiose	Belief that one has exceptional abilities, wealth, power, or fame	"I am the true President of the United States"
Erotomanic	Belief that another person is in love with oneself; often persons of fame/fortune/power are the preoccupations with erotomanic delusions	"Brittany Spears is my secret lover"
Jealous	One believes a romantic partner has been unfaithful	"My wife is cheating on me with all of my coworkers"; despite no evidence of infidelity
Somatic	Preoccupations regarding health and organ function	"There is a rat living within my stomach"
Bizarre	Clearly implausible and not understandable to peers of the same culture and do not derive from ordinary life experiences	"Aliens impregnated me in my sleep"
Nonbizarre	Situations that could be plausible	"I am an undercover CIA agent"

and mesocortical circuits of the brain as potential offenders in the development of delusions.[15] A variety of other neurobiological dysfunctions affecting different areas of the limbic system have been attributed to delusional thoughts. Dysfunction of memory processing (hippocampus) has been proposed as a cause of delusions. Researchers have identified a correlation between hypermetabolism of prefrontal and anterior cingulate regions of the brain and the development and severity of delusions.[15] Other researchers have associated the delusion of alien control with hyperactivation of the right inferior parietal lobule and cingulate gyrus.[15] Some believe that the development of delusions occurs as a means for helping to understand or better cope with any hallucinations a patient may be experiencing.[15]

SUICIDE

Psychotic symptoms can be extremely distressing to patients. Although some psychotic symptoms may improve with medical interventions, therapy, or time, often they are refractory. This leads to a life filled with turmoil, dysfunction, debilitation, multiple hospitalizations, and all too often, suicide. In the twenty-first century, more emphasis has been placed on understanding psychotic symptoms as well as improving patient care. Many cultures have come a long way in destigmatizing mental health. Yet, even now, many people are too embarrassed to reach out for help or lack the resources for adequate care. One Finnish study found that the presence of psychotic symptoms in depressed patients is a major risk factor in suicidality.[16] A meta-analysis found that when comparing depressed patients with and without psychotic features, depressed patients with psychosis have double the risk of suicide, both acutely and in lifetime risk.[2] In schizophrenia, between 5% and 13% of patients die of suicide.[17]

SUMMARY

Hallucinations, delusions, and disorganized behavior are all symptoms of psychosis, although not necessarily indicative of psychiatric illness. It is imperative to remember that *"psychosis"* is not itself a standalone disorder, rather it is a syndrome comprising of one or many symptoms; often symptoms that are quite terrifying, even debilitating for the patient. With advancements in technology and medical education, our knowledge has grown, but there is still so much to be understood. Psychosis is not exclusive to schizophrenia; a good history and pertinent examination or diagnostics may reveal an underlying condition that cannot be addressed with antipsychotics. Having a better understanding of the causes of psychotic symptoms can lead to dramatic and even life-saving improvements. A patient distressed with frequent visualizations of an abusive father is someone struggling with severe trauma and may improve with appropriate trauma therapy, avoiding the need for antipsychotics and their adverse effects. Imagine missing a brain tumor that could have been resected but was ignored due to an underlying schizophrenia diagnosis. Keeping an open and curious mind is essential in evaluation and treatment of patients who experience psychosis.

DISCLOSURE

External Advisor on PAs in Psychiatry for Alkermes.

REFERENCES

1. Nami.org. Available at: https://www.nami.org/About-Mental-Illness/Mental-Health-Conditions/Psychosis. Accessed September 22, 2020.
2. Gournellis R, Tournikioti K, Touloumi G, et al. Psychotic (delusional) depression and completed suicide: a systematic review and meta-analysis. Ann Gen Psychiatry 2018;17:39.
3. Waters F. Auditory hallucinations in adult populations 2014. Available at: https://www.psychiatrictimes.com/view/auditory-hallucinations-adult-populations. Accessed August 8, 2020.
4. Teeple RC, Caplan JP, Stern TA. Visual hallucinations: differential diagnosis and treatment. Prim Care Companion J Clin Psychiatry 2009;11(1):26–32.
5. Docherty NM, Dinzeo TJ, McCleery A, et al. Internal versus external auditory hallucinations in schizophrenia: symptom and course correlates. Cogn Neuropsychiatry 2015;20(3):187–97.
6. Sadock BJ, Sadock VA, Ruiz DP. Kaplan and Sadock's synopsis of psychiatry: behavioral sciences/clinical psychiatry. 11th edition. Baltimore, MD: Wolters Kluwer Health; 2014.
7. Waters F, Blom JD, Jardri R, et al. Auditory hallucinations, not necessarily a hallmark of psychotic disorder. Psychol Med 2018;48(4):529–36.
8. Resnick PJ, Knoll J. Faking it. How to detect malingered psychosis. Curr Psychiatr 2005;4(11):13–25.
9. Limakatso K, Bedwell GJ, Madden VJ, et al. The prevalence of phantom limb pain and associated risk factors in people with amputations: a systematic review protocol. Syst Rev 2019;8(1):17.
10. Kathirvel N, Mortimer A. Causes, diagnosis and treatment of visceral hallucinations. Prog Neurol Psychiatry 2013;17:6–10.

11. Ohayon MM. Prevalence of hallucinations and their pathological associations in the general population. Psychiatry Res 2000;97(2–3):153–64.
12. Leopold D. Distortion of olfactory perception: diagnosis and treatment. Chem Senses 2002;27(7):611–5.
13. Henkin RI, Levy LM, Fordyce A. Taste and smell function in chronic disease: a review of clinical and biochemical evaluations of taste and smell dysfunction in over 5000 patients at The Taste and Smell Clinic in Washington, DC. Am J Otolaryngol 2013;34(5):477–89.
14. Yan J. Suicide death more likely if psychosis symptoms present. Psychiatr News 2009;44(24):2–36.
15. American Psychiatric Association. Diagnostic and statistical manual of mental disorders. In: Schizophrenia spectrum and other psychotic disorders. 5th edition. American Psychiatric Association; 2013.
16. Kiran C, Chaudhury S. Understanding delusions. Ind Psychiatry J 2009; 18(1):3–18.
17. Pompili M, Amador XF, Girardi P, et al. Suicide risk in schizophrenia: learning from the past to change the future. Ann Gen Psychiatry 2007;6:10.

Cycling Without a Bike
Understanding Unipolar and Bipolar Depression

Megan E. Pater, MPAS, MA, PA-C

KEYWORDS

- Bipolar disorder • Major depressive disorder • Unipolar depression
- Cognitive impairment • Psychosocial impairment • Bipolar depression treatment

KEY POINTS

- The approach to diagnosing the correct mood disorder lies in the interview, specifically in identifying key risk factors in the setting of depression.
- Major depressive disorder and bipolar disorder have the capacity to decrease quality of life and impact functions of daily living; this is largely because of cognitive deficits and employment status.
- Treatment for bipolar depression varies, and certain medications have the potential to make the symptoms worse. Emerging adjunctive diets and therapies for unipolar and bipolar depression show promise in symptom resolution.

INTRODUCTION

Symptoms of depression can be significant in a myriad of general medical and psychological disorders. Depressed mood, sleep disturbances, loss of interest, feelings of guilt/worthlessness/hopelessness, decreased energy, decreased concentration, altered appetite, and suicidal ideation are all symptoms that describe major depressive disorder (MDD), or are they? Given this laundry list of symptoms, the differential diagnosis can be expansive, including adjustment disorder, thyroid disorder, bipolar disorder (BD), borderline personality disorder, grief, substance use disorder, MDD, and post-traumatic stress disorder (PTSD), just to name a few. Clinicians in psychiatry specialize in asking the questions and obtaining laboratory tests that provide information needed to narrow down this list. Still, information obtained during the patient encounter is often incomplete. Patients can be unreliable historians. Lack of insight, impaired recall, altered thought process, and confabulation all contribute to the complexity of psychiatry. Laboratory tests are usually only resourceful in revealing the etiology of symptoms for a handful of differentials. Imaging can reveal pathology; however, imaging does not yet contribute to any diagnostic criteria. These limitations often yield an uncertain diagnosis and can lead to improper treatment. Two common diagnoses often mistaken for each other throughout this process are MDD and BD.

Mount St Joseph University, 5701 Delhi Road, Cincinnati, OH 45233, USA
E-mail address: megan.pater@msj.edu

Physician Assist Clin 6 (2021) 505–514
https://doi.org/10.1016/j.cpha.2021.02.010
2405-7991/21/© 2021 Elsevier Inc. All rights reserved.

The two disorders are distinct, yet in the absence of mania, have many overlapping clinical presentations. A further complication is the potential to have a diagnosis of MDD with mixed features, which is new to The Diagnostic and Statistical Manual of Mental Disorders, 5th Edition (DSM-5).

Because BD tends to be more complex and has higher suicide rates, the diagnosis of MDD should be made after excluding the possibility of BD. Years of research have given more insight to these disorders including specific symptom characteristics, long-term effects, and evolving treatment regimens. These insights can help clinicians determine a more valid diagnosis, which can have considerable impact on the way clinicians implement treatment regimens and provide anticipatory guidance for patients.

ASSESSMENT

MDD is defined in the DSM-5 as five or more depressive symptoms, including depressed mood, diminished interest or pleasure in activities, weight changes, sleep disturbances, psychomotor agitation, fatigue, feelings of worthlessness or inappropriate guilt, decreased concentration, and recurrent suicidal ideation.

These symptoms are present during the same 2-week period. The symptoms must represent a change in functioning; at least one of the symptoms is either depressed mood or loss of interest in pleasure. Unipolar depression is a term used to suggest that the patient has depressive symptoms (with no specific time frame) without ever having symptoms of hypomania or mania.

The DSM-5 characterizes BP as either: bipolar I, bipolar II, or cyclothymic disorder. Bipolar I requires at least one manic episode. The manic episode may have been preceded by and may be followed by hypomanic or major depressive episodes; however hypomanic and major depressive episodes are not required for the diagnosis. A manic episode is a distinct period of abnormally and persistently elevated, expansive, or irritable mood and abnormally and persistently increased goal-directed activity or energy, lasting at least 1 week and present most of the day, nearly every day (or any duration of hospitalization is necessary). At least three of the following mania symptoms need to be present during this period:

- Inflated self-esteem or grandiosity
- Decreased need for sleep
- Flight of ideas
- More talkative than usual
- Distractibility
- Increase in goal-directed activity or psychomotor agitation
- Excessive involvement in activities that have high potential for painful consequences

Bipolar II diagnosis requires a current or past hypomanic episode and a current or past major depressive episode. Hypomania shares the same symptoms of a manic episode, but differs in timing and severity. Hypomanic episodes last at least 4 consecutive days, but do not exceed 1 week, and the episode is not severe enough to cause marked impairment in social or occupational functioning and does not necessitate hospitalization.[1]

Unipolar depression should not move BD down the list of differentials during patient assessment. There are certain symptoms that mimic depression that are predictive of BD (Table 1). Perspective studies indicate that patients with BD spend significantly more time in depression (BPII even more so than BPI) than mania/hypomania.[2] An unidentified manic or hypomanic episode and improper screening for risk factors can

Table 1
Risk factors associated with bipolar and unipolar depression

Symptoms Associated with Bipolar Depression	Symptoms Associated with Unipolar Depression
Hypersomnia	Initial insomnia/reduced sleep
Hyperphagia	Decreased appetite/weight loss
Atypical depressive features	Normal or increased activity levels
Psychomotor retardation	Somatic complaints
Psychotic features and/or pathologic guilt	Onset of first MDE >25 y
Lability of mood/manic symptoms	>6 months duration of current MDE
Onset of first MDE <25 y	Negative family history of BD
≥5 prior MDEs	
Positive family history of BD	

Data from Mitchell PB, Goodwin GM, Johnson GF, Hirschfeld RM. Diagnostic guidelines for bipolar depression: a probabilistic approach. Bipolar Disord. 2008;10(1 Pt 2):144-152.

result in years of suboptimal treatment because of an inaccurate diagnosis. In many cases, it can take up to 10 years until BD is accurately diagnosed, typically with up to four prior diagnoses.[3] Being diagnosed with MDD at a young age (<25 years) has been shown to be associated with a longer delay in BD diagnosis, especially in men. Antidepressant treatment resistance is one of the most common predictors of diagnostic conversion from MDD to BD.[4] BD patients misdiagnosed with MDD are at increased risk of attempting suicide, have significantly lower quality of life, have greater requirement for inpatient care, and account for higher total health care costs compared with BD patients who are accurately diagnosed.[5]

Screening tools for BD such as the Mood Disorder Questionnaire (MDQ) and the Hypomania Checklist (HCL-32) have reported to be useful only as aids, as they lack the specificity and sensitivity to validate the diagnosis as solitary evidence. In 2008, Mitchell and colleagues developed a "probabilistic" approach to diagnosing BD that was founded on symptoms associated with bipolar depression and unipolar depression (see **Table 1**).[6] Since then, there have been multiple studies that have verified these symptoms as risk factors for the respective mood disorder. There have also been additional risk factors found in subsequent studies that can be added to this list.

In 2010, the International Society for Bipolar Disorders also identified comorbid substance use disorder as a risk factor for bipolar depression. In 2014, Tondo and colleagues included several risk factors to their list of components that were statistically significant for BD.[7] These include attention deficit hyperactivity disorder (ADHD), BD in a first-degree relative, and mood switching during antidepressant treatment.

Later, in 2019, a study that focused on young adults suggested unipolar depression was associated with female sex and greater changes in biologic rhythm patterns when compared to bipolar depression. Additional factors (not previously stated) that correlated with bipolar depression included early childhood trauma and changes in sleep patterns (eg, day-to-night reversal).[8]

To help further differentiate from unipolar depression, comorbid personality disorders (PDs) can also serve as an indicator. A meta-analysis from 1988 to 2010 revealed that clusters B and C PDs were most prevalent in BD, specifically: paranoid, borderline, histrionic, and obsessive-compulsive PDs. Cluster C PDs (avoidant, dependent, and obsessive-compulsive) were dominant in MDD.[9]

COGNITIVE AND SOCIETAL IMPACTS

Further assisting the interview process, there are some insights relating to neuro-cognitive and psychosocial patterns that can be unveiled in patients' histories. Current research reveals some key educational points that can serve as incentives for patients to become actively involved in the awareness and recovery of their illness.

Psychomotor slowing and deficits in attention, executive function, and verbal memory have consistently been found in patients with BD.[10,11] Duration of episodes of mania or depression correlate negatively with performance on verbal memory and several executive function measurements. It has also been suggested that the number of mood episodes in BD correlates with cognitive dysfunction.[10] Additionally, euthymic patients show impairment in inhibition, task switching, verbal fluency, and visual recall.[12,13] Volkert and colleagues found that cognitive deficits in BD were associated more often with patients who reported subthreshold depressive symptoms, reduced sleep, comorbid anxiety disorder, and comorbid ADHD.

Deficits in psychomotor speed, attention, and verbal memory have been linked to sleep disturbances. Verbal memory was also influenced by prescription of antipsychotics.[12,14] This finding could be a direct result of the medication, but could also indicate that the cognitive impairments are more strongly associated with BDI, because they are more likely to be treated with an antipsychotic compared with BDII patients. There currently are inconsistent results correlating cognitive dysfunction with BDII. So far, there is evidence supporting cognitive dysfunction in BDII, but comparison studies against BDI deficits and overall severity seem to vary.[15]

In addition to cognitive defects, BDI is also associated with premature death, substance abuse, significant disability, impaired social functioning, poor work adjustment, and decreased productivity. Cognitive factors, depression, and education were found to be important factors in determining employment rate and work functioning, with cognitive factors being the most predictive.[16] In 2015, it was estimated that the cost of having BDI averaged out to be about $81,000 per individual. Further breakdown revealed that caregiving, direct health care costs, and unemployment were the biggest factors contributing toward excess costs of BDI, which were calculated to be about $48,000 per individual with BDI. These figures are likely an underestimation, as this study was not able to account for the individuals with undiagnosed BDI.[17]

In addition to BD, unipolar depression also has evidence of cognitive symptoms, sometimes appearing before the first episode. Deficits in psychomotor speed, executive function, and working memory are currently the most reported symptoms. These deficits, in addition to impaired divided attention, have been correlated to significant work impairment and potential loss of employment.[18] Unipolar depression has been shown to have a detrimental effect on education, work or school attendance, and employment. The severity and duration of depressive episodes correlated with an increase in work days missed and subsequently lower employment rates.[16] In addition to the cognitive deficits mentioned, functional recovery is impaired by difficulty concentrating and indecisiveness. There is evidence that suggests improvement in these symptoms with an antidepressant; however, most studies are inconclusive about the magnitude of improvement and factors that contribute to residual symptoms.[18] The importance of early intervention and treatment adherence becomes not only a matter of symptom control, but a potentially important intervention to protect against functional decline.

Impaired psychosocial functioning has various manifestations; over time, some common themes have emerged. Both MDD and BD patients showed neglect in household chores, poor work performance, impairments in relationships, and overall dissatisfaction with their quality of life. Improvements in all areas were seen after 6 weeks of pharmacologic treatment. Despite the improvements, occupational and relational difficulties had the least impressive magnitude of enhancement and often persisted for most patients.[11]

TREATMENT

Antidepressants are still the mainstay of pharmacologic interventions for treating MDD. The STAR*D trial assessed remission rates with antidepressant treatment. Of the patients enrolled in the study, 36% went into remission with citalopram alone (level 1). Of those who moved onto level 2 (indicating symptoms were unresolved in level 1), 30.6% had success after altering their treatment (**Fig. 1**).

Although 67% of participants remitted, about half relapsed by 1 year follow-up. These results illustrate the unfortunate challenge of sustaining remission while treating MDD, and they imply that modulating monoamine neurotransmission alone is not sufficient for long-term remission in most patients.[19,20] Depression is usually considered resistant or refractory when at least 2 appropriate trials of antidepressants from different pharmacologic classes fail to produce significant improvements. It is estimated that up to 15% of patients treated for unipolar depression will fall into the category of treatment-resistant depression (TRD). Higher prevalence of TRD is often reported because of failures in adequate screening for BD and hypothyroidism. Additionally, falsely elevated rates of TRD may be reflective of inadequate compliance with medication.[21]

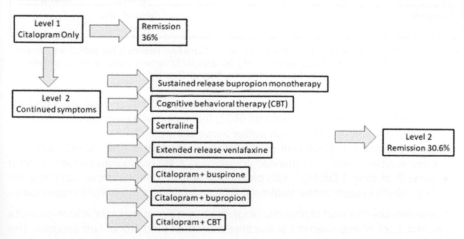

Fig. 1. STAR*D trial (level 1 and 2). (*Data From* Friborg O, Martinsen EW, Martinussen M, Kaiser S, Overgård KT, Rosenvinge JH. Comorbidity of personality disorders in mood disorders: a meta-analytic review of 122 studies from 1988 to 2010. J Affect Disord. 2014;152-154:1-1.)

The 2018, the Canadian Network for Mood and Anxiety Treatments (CANMAT) and International Society for Bipolar Disorders (ISBD) released guidelines for the management of patients with BD. Recommendations are based on line-of-treatment ratings that are formulated from level-of-evidence ratings (**Table 2**):

Table 2
.2018 hierarchical rankings of first and second-line treatments recommended for management of bipolar depression[3]

Medication (Target Doses/Serum Levels)	BDI: Acute Depression	BDI: Maintenance for Prevention of Any Mood Episode	BDII: Acute Depression	BDII: Maintenance Treatment
Quetiapine (300 mg/d)	First-line, level 1	First-line, level 1	First-line, level 1	First-line, level 1
Lurasidone + lithium/divalproex	First-line, level 1			
Lithium (0.8–1.2 mEq/L)	First-line, level 2	First-line, level 1	Second-line, level 2	First-line, level 2
Lamotrigine (200 mg/d)	First-line, level 2	First-line, level 1	Second-line, level 2	First-line level 2
Divalproex	Second-line, level 2	Second-line, level 1		
SSRIs/bupropion (adj)	Second-line, level 2			
Cariprazine	Second-line, level 1			
Olanzapine-fluoxetine	Second-line, level 2			
Venlafaxine			Second-line, level 2	Second-line, level 2
Sertraline			Second-line, level 2	

Data From Yatham LN, Kennedy SH, Parikh SV, et al. Canadian Network for Mood and Anxiety Treatments (CANMAT) and International Society for Bipolar Disorders (ISBD) 2018 guidelines for the management of patients with bipolar disorder. Bipolar Disord.

- Level 1: a meta-analysis with narrow confidence interval or replicated double-blind (DB), randomized control trial (RCT) that includes a placebo or active control comparison (n ≥30 in each active treatment arm)
- Level 2: a meta-analysis with wide confidence interval or one DB RCT with placebo or active control comparison condition (n ≥30 in each active treatment arm)
- Level 3: at least 1 DB RCT with placebo or active control comparison condition (n = 10–29 in each active treatment arm) or health system administrative data

Two weeks after the start of pharmacologic therapy is a reasonable time to re-evaluate symptoms. Lack of improvement at this time is a robust predictor of nonresponse. The exception to this theory is when using lamotrigine, because of the slow-titration recommended to ensure safety from potential emerging adverse effects. Antidepressants were discouraged as monotherapy for BDI depression because of the possibility of treatment-emergent mania. Aripiprazole and ziprasidone were 2 atypical antipsychotics that failed to show significant efficacy in BDI depression. There are no first-line psychosocial treatment options for acute bipolar depression. Psychoeducation and psychosocial strategies are recommended in addition to medication to promote medication adherence, reduce residual symptoms and suicidal behavior, help identify early signs of relapse, and support functional recovery.[3]

A recent meta-analysis in 2020 revealed slightly different pharmacologic monotherapy treatments for bipolar depression than previously mentioned. The study's analysis of the most effective atypical antipsychotics, antidepressants, and mood stabilizers are summarized in **Table 3**. It appeared that the antidepressants listed did not produce a significant increase in the rate of treatment-emergent mania. This certainly challenges previous data findings and historic wisdom; however, it can be viewed as a compelling option when the diagnosis between MDD and BD is uncertain. Escitalopram, phenelzine, carbamazepine, sertraline, lithium, paroxetine, aripiprazole, gabapentin, and ziprasidone were ineffective compared with placebo in treatment of bipolar depression.[22]

Table 3
.2020 most effective monotherapy pharmacologic treatments for bipolar depression[22]

Atypical Antipsychotics	Antidepressants	Mood Stabilizers
Cariprazine	Tranylcypromine	Lamotrigine
Lurasidone	Fluoxetine	Divalproex
Quetiapine	Venlafaxine	
Olanzapine	Imipramine	

Data From Bahji A, Ermacora D, Stephenson C, Hawken ER, Vazquez G. Comparative efficacy and tolerability of pharmacological treatments for the treatment of acute bipolar depression: A systematic review and network meta-analysis. J Affect Disord. 2020;269:154-184.

Adjunctive treatment options for MDD and bipolar depression are continuing to expand as the understanding of the pathophysiology behind the disease states improve. The effects of omega (n)-3 and omega (n)-6 polyunsaturated fatty acids (PUFA) are being investigated as key players in the neuro-inflammatory process that has been linked to BD.[23] Research has shown improvement of symptoms in bipolar depression when using omega (n)-3 as adjunctive treatment.[24] Because of the properties of each fatty acid, a high intake of omega (n)-3 in conjunction with a low intake of omega (n)-6 is the approach that many researchers are investigating for an even greater benefit to symptoms in bipolar depression.[23]

The Mediterranean diet is founded on consumption of plant-based foods such as vegetables, fruits, whole grains, beans, nuts, seeds, olive oil, and limited intake of red meat. This diet, in addition to exercising, has been shown to improve depressive symptoms in MDD[25,26] and implies (although not specifically studied) benefits for BD also. Adhering to a Mediterranean diet and an exercise program has further benefits in reducing stroke and cognitive impairment.[27]

In addition to diet, specific types of psychotherapies are emerging as beneficial for MDD and BD. Psychodynamic therapy was recently demonstrated to be as effective as cognitive behavioral therapy in reducing depressive symptoms during treatment of MDD. Despite having additional options for nonpharmacological therapy, depression still remains to be a difficult-to-treat disorder, and the overall efficacy of psychotherapy for depression needs to be improved.[28]

Developing therapeutic approaches for BD have shown promise, specifically in regard to interpersonal and social rhythm therapy (IPSRT). This type of therapy acknowledges how alterations in daily routines, psychosocial stressors, and life events may place substantial stress on the body's capacity to maintain stable biologic rhythms, and therefore make someone with BD more prone to episodes of depression or mania.[29] IPSRT is founded on the idea that recurrence of mood episodes in BD occurs most often when there is nonadherence to medication, presence of a stressful life event, and disruptions in social rhythms.

With this knowledge, IPSRT is geared toward stabilizing patients' routines while simultaneously improving the quality of their interpersonal relationships and their performance of key social roles. IPSRT is typically implemented in 4 stages over 24 sessions within a 9-month period of time. IPRST can be used as an intervention method of treatment in BD regardless of current mood status. So far, this type of therapy has been proven to be beneficial in regulating circadian rhythms by normalizing daily rhythms, thus preventing relapsing moods and reducing acute affective symptoms. Currently, good supporting evidence exists that IPRST can be effective for treating BDII as monotherapy[30]; however this type of therapy is still considered third-line adjunctive treatment for acute and maintenance depression in BDI because of limited level 2 evidence.[3]

SUMMARY

Bipolar depression and MDD have many overlapping symptoms that often result in misdiagnosis. Using a probabilistic approach aids in determining a more valid diagnosis that can further ensure proper treatment. Declines in quality of life, most often marked by cognitive deficits, is seen in both MDD and BD. Emerging research about pharmacologic treatment for these disorders is slightly conflicting; however, advancements in adjunctive therapy concerning diet and psychotherapy leave reason to be hopeful about an improved long-term prognosis.

DISCLOSURE

The author has nothing to disclose.

REFERENCES

1. Diagnostic and statistical manual of mental disorders: DSM-5. 5th edition. Arlington (VA): American Psychiatric Publishing; 2013.
2. Manning JS. Burden of illness in bipolar depression. Prim Care Companion J Clin Psychiatry 2005;7(6):259–67.
3. Yatham LN, Kennedy SH, Parikh SV, et al. Canadian Network for Mood and Anxiety Treatments (CANMAT) and International Society for Bipolar Disorders (ISBD) 2018 guidelines for the management of patients with bipolar disorder. Bipolar Disord 2018;20(2):97–170.
4. Fritz K, Russell AMT, Allwang C, et al. Is a delay in the diagnosis of bipolar disorder inevitable? Bipolar Disord 2017;19(5):396–400.
5. Schaffer A, Cairney J, Veldhuizen S, et al. A population-based analysis of distinguishers of bipolar disorder from major depressive disorder. J Affect Disord 2010; 125(1–3):103–10.
6. Mitchell PB, Goodwin GM, Johnson GF, et al. Diagnostic guidelines for bipolar depression: a probabilistic approach. Bipolar Disord 2008;10(1 Pt 2):144–52.
7. Tondo L, Visioli C, Preti A, et al. Bipolar disorders following initial depression: modeling predictive clinical factors. J Affect Disord 2014;167:44–9.
8. Patella AM, Jansen K, Cardoso TA, et al. Clinical features of differential diagnosis between unipolar and bipolar depression in a drug-free sample of young adults. J Affect Disord 2019;243:103–7.

9. Friborg O, Martinsen EW, Martinussen M, et al. Comorbidity of personality disorders in mood disorders: a meta-analytic review of 122 studies from 1988 to 2010. J Affect Disord 2014;152-154:1–11.

10. López-Jaramillo C, Lopera-Vásquez J, Gallo A, et al. Effects of recurrence on the cognitive performance of patients with bipolar I disorder: implications for relapse prevention and treatment adherence. Bipolar Disord 2010;12(5):557–67.

11. Xu G, Lin K, Rao D, et al. Neuropsychological performance in bipolar I, bipolar II and unipolar depression patients: a longitudinal, naturalistic study. J Affect Disord 2012;136(3):328–39.

12. Pålsson E, Figueras C, Johansson AG, et al. Neurocognitive function in bipolar disorder: a comparison between bipolar I and II disorder and matched controls. BMC Psychiatry 2013;13:165.

13. Robinson LJ, Thompson JM, Gallagher P, et al. A meta-analysis of cognitive deficits in euthymic patients with bipolar disorder. J Affect Disord 2006;93(1–3): 105–15.

14. Volkert J, Kopf J, Kazmaier J, et al. Evidence for cognitive subgroups in bipolar disorder and the influence of subclinical depression and sleep disturbances. Eur Neuropsychopharmacol 2015;25(2):192–202.

15. Solé B, Martínez-Arán A, Torrent C, et al. Are bipolar II patients cognitively impaired? A systematic review. Psychol Med 2011;41(9):1791–803.

16. Gilbert E, Marwaha S. Predictors of employment in bipolar disorder: a systematic review. J Affect Disord 2013;145(2):156–64.

17. Cloutier M, Greene M, Guerin A, et al. The economic burden of bipolar I disorder in the United States in 2015. J Affect Disord 2018;226:45–51.

18. Trivedi MH, Greer TL. Cognitive dysfunction in unipolar depression: implications for treatment. J Affect Disord 2014;152-154:19–27.

19. Rush AJ, Trivedi MH, Wisniewski SR, et al. Acute and longer-term outcomes in depressed outpatients requiring one or several treatment steps: a STAR*D report. Am J Psychiatry 2006;163(11):1905–17.

20. Frye MA, Helleman G, McElroy SL, et al. Correlates of treatment-emergent mania associated with antidepressant treatment in bipolar depression. Am J Psychiatry 2009;166(2):164–72.

21. Berlim MT, Turecki G. Definition, assessment, and staging of treatment-resistant refractory major depression: a review of current concepts and methods. Can J Psychiatry 2007;52(1):46–54.

22. Bahji A, Ermacora D, Stephenson C, et al. Comparative efficacy and tolerability of pharmacological treatments for the treatment of acute bipolar depression: A systematic review and network meta-analysis. J Affect Disord 2020;269:154–84.

23. Saunders EF, Ramsden CE, Sherazy MS, et al. Reconsidering dietary polyunsaturated fatty acids in bipolar disorder: a translational picture. J Clin Psychiatry 2016;77(10):e1342–7.

24. Sarris J, Mischoulon D, Schweitzer I. Omega-3 for bipolar disorder: meta-analyses of use in mania and bipolar depression. J Clin Psychiatry 2012; 73(1):81–6.

25. Jacka FN, O'Neil A, Opie R, et al. A randomised controlled trial of dietary improvement for adults with major depression (the 'SMILES' trial). BMC Med 2017;15(1):23 [published correction appears in BMC Med. 2018;16(1):236].

26. Masana MF, Haro JM, Mariolis A, et al. Mediterranean diet and depression among older individuals: The multinational MEDIS study. Exp Gerontol 2018;110:67–72.

27. Psaltopoulou T, Sergentanis TN, Panagiotakos DB, et al. Mediterranean diet, stroke, cognitive impairment, and depression: a meta-analysis. Ann Neurol 2013;74(4):580–91.
28. Driessen E, Van HL, Peen J, et al. Cognitive-behavioral versus psychodynamic therapy for major depression: secondary outcomes of a randomized clinical trial. J Consult Clin Psychol 2017;85(7):653–63.
29. Frank E, Swartz HA, Boland E. Interpersonal and social rhythm therapy: an intervention addressing rhythm dysregulation in bipolar disorder. Dialogues Clin Neurosci 2007;9(3):325–32.
30. Swartz HA, Levenson JC, Frank E. Psychotherapy for bipolar II disorder: the role of interpersonal and social rhythm therapy. Prof Psychol Res Pr 2012;43(2): 145–53.

Overwhelmed by Bodily Sensations
Understanding Somatic Symptom Disorders

Phyllis R. Peterson, PA-C, MPAS, CAQpsy[a,b,*]

KEYWORDS

- Somatic symptom disorder • Illness anxiety disorder
- Functional neurologic symptom disorder • Factitious disorder
- Psychological factors affecting a medical condition

INTRODUCTION

Somatic symptom disorders are poorly understood, commonly misdiagnosed, and thus left untreated. This is costly to both the patient and the health care system. The *Diagnostic and Statistical Manual of Mental Disorders* (DSM) historically has given short shrift to somatic disorders often combining it with other diagnoses. However, in the most recent version, the fifth edition (DSM 5), somatic disorders are now grouped together in a separate section.[1] The newest classification system includes diagnostic criteria, differentials, and epidemiologic data. Even with this separation into its own category, there are areas of confusion clinically and it is the author's hope to help clarify these disorders through systematic and stepwise evaluation and management.

HISTORY

The history of somatization and somatic disorders is tied to the history of anxiety in medicine, neurology, philosophy, and psychology. Anxiety was differentiated from mood or sadness by Greek and Latin philosophers and physicians.[2] Ancient scholars believed in the mind/body connection and felt a disruption in this connection led to disorders. There were efforts to explain both the source of disruption and methods of treatment. The Latin orator, Cicero (106 BC to 43 BC), writing of his daughter's death, postulated that a troubled mind produces worry and anxiety and identified "worry and anxiety" as an illness. He proposed stoicism as treatment. Even today, stoicism is a major tenet of mindful meditation and a mainstay in modern cognitive behavioral therapy (CBT).[3]

The Epicurean school of philosophy theorized that a fear of death was the source of unhappiness.[2] Egyptian physicians noted more physical symptoms in men than

[a] NP PA Post Graduate Psychiatry Program, Texas Tech University Health Sciences Center, Lubbock, TX, USA; [b] Psychiatric PA Services, Leander, TX, USA
* 2321 Broken Wagon Drive, Leander, TX 78641.
E-mail address: psychpa@hotmail.com

Physician Assist Clin 6 (2021) 515–526
https://doi.org/10.1016/j.cpha.2021.02.011
2405-7991/21/© 2021 Elsevier Inc. All rights reserved.
physicianassistant.theclinics.com

women. They felt women had a "floating uterus" and this protected women from anxiety.[4]

Later, anxiety was not viewed as a separate psychiatric illness, but included in the diagnoses of melancholy and depression. In the 18th century, Robert Burton used the term "panophobia" for anxiety.[2] In the early 20th century, Robert Kraepelin, often called the father of modern scientific psychiatry, described anxiety as a frequent symptom of other disorders and a descriptor in bipolar disorder.[2]

The DSM-1 was mainly influenced by psychoanalytical theory. It included many terms for anxiety coined by Sigmund Freud: psychoneurotic objective anxiety, neurotic anxiety, and unconscious neurosis.[2,5] By the publication of the third edition of the DSM, anxiety was divided into panic and generalized anxiety. This split was due to evidence that imipramine showed an ability to block panic attacks but not generalized anxiety (also referred to as phobic anxiety).[6] The DSM III changes also reflected the psychiatric trend to view mental illnesses as arising from brain chemistry with pharmacologic rather than psychoanalysis treatment.[4,6] The classification of anxiety disorders was not changed significantly in fourth edition of the DSM, although somatization was added.[7] In the 1990s, the thinking was that somatization was a method used by patients, purposefully or not, to produce symptoms for secondary gain. These symptoms could include the benefits of the "sick role," manipulation of others or the medical and legal systems, and disability. The attention was more on "unexplained medical symptoms" and malingering.[8]

SOMATIC SYMPTOM AND RELATED DISORDERS

The DSM-5 introduced Somatic Symptom and Related Disorders as a separate chapter and defined somatic disorders as physical signs and symptoms that cause distress and/or dysfunction (**Box 1**).[1]

The 7 disorders within the somatic chapter are linked with common features of physical symptoms predominated by worry, attention, and behaviors that are distressing or result in significant disruption of daily life.[1] Although any 1 somatic symptom may not be continuously present (specific symptoms can be transient), the state of being symptomatic is persistent. Persistence is defined as 6 months or more.[1]

The somatic symptoms and related disorders category combined DSM IV somatization disorder, hypochondriasis, pain disorder, and undifferentiated somatoform disorders with a new grouping using common clinical features.[1] This change was a reaction to the confusion and overlap previous DSM versions had caused for primary

---

Box 1
Somatic symptoms and related disorders as listed in the DSM 5[1]

Somatic symptom disorder

Illness anxiety disorder

Conversion disorder (functional neurologic symptom disorder)

Psychological factors affecting other medical conditions

Factitious disorder imposed on self or imposed on another

Other specific somatic symptom and related disorder

Unspecified somatic symptom and related disorder

Adapted from American Psychiatric Association: Diagnostic and Statistical Manual of Mental Disorders, Fifth Edition. American Psychiatric Association; 2013.

care providers.[5] Because somatic disorders are mainly encountered in primary care ($\leq$30% of visits) and emergency departments (ED) rather than psychiatric ambulatory settings, the focus on identification for primary care providers is imperative.[3,4] The DSM 5 offers a more clinically relevant classification of somatic illness with a concentration on symptoms and the distress they cause. This new somatic chapter also integrates our increasing knowledge of genetics, neurobiology, pathophysiology, and the variation of biologic vulnerability and sensitizing events.[1,5]

Many providers and medical personnel see somatic patients as "problems." This conceptualization can damage the patient's trust in medicine and can affect patient self-esteem. The issues of repeated evaluations, multiple medications, and a myriad of laboratory tests and procedures can cause iatrogenic harm to the patient as well as increased costs to the health system.[5] A simple paradigm shift is often needed with the understanding that somatic disorders symptoms are not conscious or "made up," but instead are unconscious expressions of real pain and suffering. If one approaches this case as intriguing and able to be solved, rather than a problem, a more appropriate evaluation and management can be ordered, and the results evaluated. This practice alleviates distress for the patient as well as providers.

Prior nomenclature and approaches have been stigmatizing to patients, confusing to providers, and reinforcing an approach of nontreatment and avoidance for this patient population. In recent years, there have been efforts to standardize criteria, educate providers, and develop guidelines for evaluation and treatment of somatic disorders in the primary care setting.[4]

The exact pathophysiologic cause of somatic disorders is unclear, but there is evidence of neurobiological, neuroplastic, and genetic involvement. Liu and colleagues[9] reviewed the interaction of serotonergic and noradrenergic systems in the central nervous system and peripheral levels. This interaction was mainly viewed through the actions of various antidepressants on somatic systems. There is a need for further study in determining how mediation of pain and other somatic symptoms differs from or is similar to other psychiatric illnesses.[9]

Precipitating and predictive factors include psychological distress resulting from abuse and trauma interacting with socioeconomic, cultural, and spiritual influences. One area of controversy is that many psychiatric illnesses share the same or similar brain structure changes and predisposing factors and risks. A large portion of patients who meet criteria for a somatic disorder also have medical and psychiatric comorbidities (**Table 1**). This factor makes sorting out the specific etiology difficult.[1,4,5]

Data on somatic disorders are limited because this is a new separate category. Before the publication of the DMS 5, somatic disorders were listed in multiple areas of the DSM IV. It is estimated that somatic disorders occur in 5% to 7% of the population.[5] However, it is believed that primary care rates are higher, as are incidence rates of women to men (10:1).[5] The onset of somatic disease usually occurs in the 20s, although symptoms can present at any age, including in the elderly ($\geq$65 years of age).[5] Somatic disorder may be underdiagnosed in older individuals because increased complaints are seen as part of aging, in this situation the extent of the worry should be considered.[1] The triggering event is thought to be an abnormally heightened sensitivity to bodily functions and a tendency to interpret them as illness related.

Higher incidence occurs in those with[1,3,5]:

- Less education
- Lower incomes
- History of trauma from child abuse
- History of adverse events

Table 1
Differentiating somatic symptoms and related disorders[1,4,5,10]

Disorder	Motivation	Symptoms	Thoughts/Behaviors
Somatic symptom disorder	Unconscious somatic sensations heightened	Bodily symptoms causing distress Seek relief of symptoms	Abnormal thoughts, feelings, behaviors about signs and symptoms
Illness anxiety disorder	Unconscious	Worry/fear of illness with few or minor signs and symptoms Seek confirmation	Preoccupation having an illness or getting sick
Conversion disorder	Unconscious	Neurologic (motor or sensory) symptoms or loss of function Seek return to function	Indication of incompatibility with neurologic disorder
Psychological factors affecting medical condition	Unconscious or conscious	Varies with disorders	Interferes with treatment, progress
Factitious disorder (imposed on self or others)	Conscious	Varies with symptom or disorder imposed	Indications of deception No external gain

- New or chronic illness

There seems to be a genetic and environmental component leading to increased sensitivity to discomfort as well.[1] Although there are differences in symptoms and presentations among various cultures, the features of increased anxiety, depression, and dysfunction are common to all.[1,3]

In 2020, the coronavirus disease 2019 pandemic increased the presentation of somatic symptoms.[11] More recently, Shevlin and colleagues[11] studied anxiety and somatic symptoms in the UK. They found that people with higher rates of anxiety regarding coronavirus disease 2019 had higher rates of somatic symptoms, especially pain, fatigue, and gastrointestinal distress.[11] Data from the 2003 severe acute respiratory syndrome epidemic showed that there were increased levels of anxiety, depression and somatization, which increased with more time spent in quarantine.[12]

TREATMENT OF SOMATIC AND RELATED DISORDERS

After evaluation and diagnosis, treatment begins with the sharing of the diagnosis. Leaving the diagnosis unsaid is not only inappropriate, it leaves patients feeling they are dismissed and/or viewed with suspicion.[5] It is important to confirm a diagnosis and the concept that it is likely brain based. Many practitioners use the hardware/software explanation. The brain (hardware) shows no abnormality in common testing. However, the brain circuits or messaging (software), are malfunctioning.[10]

To decrease nonadherence and mistrust, it is necessary patients feel listened to and their feelings acknowledged.[5] All staff (medical and office) must understand the legitimacy of symptoms and the appropriate approach. Patients should be told their somatic disorder is likely influenced by many factors: stress and coping mechanisms, illness beliefs, and exacerbated sensitivity to bodily functions. Patients should be told that there will be a waxing and waning of the symptoms over time. After an evaluation and diagnosis, the treatment is multifaceted, collaborative, and individualized. The goal of this approach is to decrease symptoms, distress, and medical service costs. One of the most effective methods is the CARE MD approach[4,5] (**Table 2**).

Patients are often referred to the psychiatric consultation and liaison service after extensive in-patient evaluation to rule out medical causes. A treatment plan that suits the patient's needs but includes frequent scheduled visits, possible CBT, and enforces the need for communication and collaboration among providers must be developed. Collaboration between all providers can assure coordination, provide support between providers and by extension, the patient. There may be need for more intense psychodynamic therapy, that is, eye movement desensitization and reprocessing, to address the primary psychopathology, which can be mood disorders, personality disorders, and/or trauma. Ongoing motivational interviewing and patient education can assist in setting patient goals, assessing progress and changing behavioral learning. There is evidence for use of virtual reality.[13]

SOMATIC SYMPTOM DISORDER

The criteria for somatic symptom disorder includes having 1 or more symptoms present for 6 or more months that interfere with daily function. Patients may experience excessive thoughts, feelings, and behaviors out of proportion to seriousness of physical symptoms.[1]

The presentation of somatic symptom disorder varies in terms of both the types and number of symptoms. Common somatic symptom disorder symptoms involve pain, fatigue, gastrointestinal, genitourinary, cardiovascular, dermatologic, and/or neurologic presentations. There is often a waxing and waning of the number and intensity of symptoms, although 1 particular symptom is the most severe. Worry is often out of proportion with thoughts, feelings, and behaviors draining the patient's time, relationships, and ability to function.[1] The feeling of being "ill" becomes a central characteristic of the patient's life. These patients may have a history of frequent evaluations, tests, consultations, and even procedures. Various studies of unexplained medical symptoms show that 50% to 75% of those affected show improvements over time, and about 10% to 30% deteriorate.[14]

Table 2 CARE MD approach[5]		
C	Consultation/ collaboration	Work collaboratively with psychiatry and therapist (CBT)
A	Assessment	Rule-out other medical and psychiatric diseases
R	Regular visits	Schedule limited time, regular visits, focus on coping vs cure
E	Empathy	Listen, accept, and reassure that feelings are real
M	Medical/psychiatric interface	Focus on mind–body connections, avoid saying "all in your head" or "you have no medical disease" or "you are exaggerating or making up"[a]
D	Do no harm	Avoid testing, referrals to subspecialist reassure known medical illnesses were ruled-out

[a] Note this applies to all staff who contact patient in any manner.

Somatic symptom disorder must be differentiated from a medical illness, anxiety, panic, depression, delusional disorder, body dysmorphic disorder, obsessive-compulsive disorder, illness anxiety, and conversion disorder.[1] The diagnosis of a medical condition will negate the somatic symptom disorder diagnosis, namely, irritable bowel syndrome or fibromyalgia. The initial assessment for somatic symptom disorder requires both medical and psychiatric causes to be addressed and treated. Often, differentiation between other diagnosis and somatic symptom disorder can be accomplished simply with a good history, because these patients have undergone significant physical examinations as well as laboratory, neurologic, and radiologic testing.[1,5]

Most patients welcome the diagnosis of somatic symptom disorder with its explanation of the mind–body connection and the neurobiological evidence of heightened sensitivity to normal bodily sensations. Although this explanation provides reassurance for many patients, some patients are less accepting. Interactions between providers, staff, and patients must always portray acceptance and support. Collaboration with mental health experts is paramount. Studies show methods to decrease symptoms often involve a multifaceted treatment plan that can include CBT.[5] A meta-analysis of mindfulness-based therapy showed improvement of symptoms severity, depression and anxiety for up to 2 years with significant cost effectiveness.[15]

On-going treatment monitoring includes quarterly Patient Health Questionnaire-15 or the Somatic Symptom Scale-8 or the Well-being Scale. The Patient Health Questionnaire-15 version is preferred over the shorter Patient Health Questionnaire-9 owing to the addition of questions regarding menstrual issues, headache, and/or pain.

Medication can be helpful. Frequently there are comorbidities, especially major depressive disorder or post-traumatic stress disorder, that guide pharmacotherapy. On its own, somatic symptom disorder has shown improvement with 2 antidepressants, fluoxetine and amitriptyline. Both medications have shown decreases in fatigue, morning stiffness, improved sleep, pain tender points, and overall well-being.[4,16] Although there are no controlled trials, similar antidepressants may also be effective and may be more appropriate depending on patient preference, history, and comorbidities.[16,17] Trials showing effectiveness and tolerability of St John's wart in comparison to placebo were low quality and self-reported.[18] There is no evidence for monoamines inhibitors, bupropion, antiepileptic, or antipsychotic medications and these agents should be avoided.[17] Caution is advised when combining antidepressants with other medications, especially cancer medications, antineoplastic drugs, and birth control pills.[19]

ILLNESS ANXIETY DISORDER

Previously referred to as hypochondriasis, illness anxiety disorder is fear, worry, self-checking, and preoccupation regarding an illness. Thoughts and related behaviors can cause significant dysfunction. Differential diagnoses include medical illness, adjustment disorder, anxiety, obsessive compulsive disorder, somatic symptom disorder, major depressive disorder, and psychotic disorders.[1] There are 2 major types of illness anxiety disorder: care seeking (more common) and care avoiding. Criteria are similar to somatic symptom disorder: symptoms present for 6 months or more and are not caused by a medical condition. The prevalence is difficult to ascertain, but is thought to be between 0.04% and 4.50%.[20] The high costs attributed to this disorder include higher rates of health care services, lost workdays, and disability benefits.

In illness anxiety disorder, the patient will present with complaints of a specific disorder. Although the symptoms may be minimal or nonexistent, the concern, the fear, and preoccupation of illness prevail. The patient has likely spent time researching the disease state and develops symptoms in response. Because much of the research is done via the internet, this is often called cyberchondria. Patients are rarely reassured by medical explanations or negative testing. Their attentions to bodily functions increase their anxiety and fear and exacerbates their perceived illness. Thus, it becomes a circular issue.[20]

As with somatic symptom disorder, many of these patients have undergone significant medical evaluations and testing leading to the need for psychiatric evaluation. Treatment using the CARE MD guidelines along with collaboration among practitioners is important. Time-limited appointments with primary care should be scheduled. Medications can be helpful, although evidence is minimal. Double-blinded, controlled studies of fluoxetine and paroxetine have demonstrated efficacy over placebo, although much of the treatment response was before the reclassification of illness anxiety disorder within the DSM 5.[20] One long-term study of patients taking selective serotonin reuptake inhibitors found that 60% of patients no longer met the criteria for illness anxiety disorder at 8 years.[17] Medications in combination with CBT were effective, but benzodiazepines and antipsychotic medications should be avoided.[20] Documentation and communication with all providers should include cautions regarding unnecessary testing and evaluation while noting that concurrent medical illness can occur. Use of scales like Whitely Index (http://www.nvcbt.com/self-help-quizzes/health-anxiety-self-assessment/) or Illness Attitudes Scale are useful for evaluation and progression of illness anxiety disorder (https://www.kcl.ac.uk/ioppn/depts/psychology/research/ResearchGroupings/CADAT/Links/Illness-Attitudes-Questionnaire-(PDF).pdf).

CONVERSION DISORDER (FUNCTIONAL NEUROLOGIC SYMPTOM DISORDER)

Conversion disorder and functional neurologic symptom disorder are used interchangeably in the DSM-5 and most literature. Conversion disorder involves an alteration or loss of voluntarily controlled sensory or motor function incompatible with a known neurologic disorder, such as stroke, seizure, or tremor. The sensory and motor symptoms must cause distress, impairment, or dysfunction. Although conversion disorder is most commonly used, the term functional neurologic symptom disorder considers the causative factors; in other words, the incompatibility of physical symptoms and any known neurologic disorder.[1] There are 2 large groups: motor symptoms and sensory symptoms, although these groupings are not always discrete.

The DSM-5 criteria call for a specification of type (weakness, paralysis, movement, gait, sensation, or special senses) as well as acute versus persistent and if psychological stress is present.[1] Historically the phenomenon of *la belle indifference* (inappropriately complacent attitude toward their condition and physical symptoms) was thought to be pathognomonic for functional neurologic symptom disorder; however, in the DSM 5, it is not included in the criteria.[1]

The neurobiological theory is that motor areas are hypoactive or disconnected with areas that select or inhibit movement. The evaluation should specify the incompatibility symptoms. Common clues in the neurologic examination include the Hoover sign (a variation of muscle tone between 2 tests), nonanatomic sensory loss, exaggerated compensatory movement (flailing) and a mismatch between physical tests (ie, weak plantar flexion on bed but able to toe walk). With tremors, the patient may show differences in tremors if distracted or during changes in positioning.[21] With seizure presentation, there may be a lack of postictal confusion or the patient has the ability to recall activity and conversations during the seizure. The patient may respond to external stimuli and resist outside attempts to lift their eyelids. There may be a fluctuating course or non–seizure-type movements such as pelvic thrusting or side-to-side movements.[21]

The onset of conversion is typically acute, with or without psychological or physical stressors. There is often a repetitive or ongoing course throughout the patient's lifespan. The incidence in women is 2 to 3 times higher.[1,22] The prevalence is unknown; however, conversion is more commonly seen in primary care and/or ED. ED presentation is often due to stroke-like symptoms or nonepileptic seizures.[20] Conversion disorder (functional neurologic symptom disorder) accounts for 5% of referrals to neurology.[1] The differentials for conversion disorder (functional neurologic symptom disorder) include neurologic disorder, somatic symptom disorder, major depressive disorder, factitious disorder, panic disorder, and dissociative disorder. Conversion disorder (functional neurologic symptom disorder) commonly presents concurrently with anxiety, panic, and/or depression.[1]

To identify incidence and presentation, the research group from Cambridge reviewed 300 patients who presented to the ED with motor-only symptoms.[23] The most common complaint was weakness. Common demographics included female sex, married, prior employment, more physical health conditions (on average) and lower rates of prior psychiatric hospitalizations. Interestingly, history of abuse was not more frequent compared with other psychiatric conditions.[23] Positive prognostic factors for conversion disorder (functional neurologic symptom disorder) include acceptance of the diagnosis and a short duration of symptoms. The prognosis can be affected adversely by personality traits or disorders, abuse, a previous history of functional neurologic symptom disorder, a family history of functional neurologic symptom disorder, and/or stressful life events. Patients with epilepsy may also have nonepileptic seizures.

Treatment should follow CARE MD guide with buy-in among all practitioners and medical/clerical staff. Physical therapy or occupational therapy using treatment strategies to decrease attention to the abnormal movement specifically not using supportive devices is well-established. The use of CBT and motivational interviewing (to increase engagement in treatment) is also well-established.[5] There are also early positive findings for the use of virtual reality.[14]

PSYCHOLOGICAL FACTORS AFFECTING OTHER MEDICAL CONDITIONS

The cornerstone of the diagnosis of physiologic factors affecting other medical conditions requires a confirmed medical diagnosis but with behaviors or psychological factors interfering with that illness causing disability, harm, or death. The criteria include a lack of treatment progress, exacerbation of the medical condition, interference with treatment, and/or additional risk adding to the pathophysiology. The underlying medical condition may be an illness or injury, acute or chronic, and includes such disparate diagnoses as pain, fatigue, irritable bowel syndrome, headache, cancer, diabetes, or cardiac disease. The psychological effects and behaviors cannot be due to a secondary mental disorder; however, they may be comorbid, such as depression with cardiac disease.[1]

The etiology is often influenced by health beliefs, life events, the provider–patient relationship, communication, family, and/or gender roles. Although culture can play a role, if the belief or practice does not interfere with medical management, it does not qualify. The disorders can occur anytime during the lifespan. Differential diagnoses include psychiatric conditions caused by a medical condition, somatic symptom disorder, illness anxiety disorder, and/or adjustment disorder. The prevalence is unknown, although third-party payers report that this disorder occurs more often than somatic symptom disorder.[1]

In psychiatric conditions caused by a medical illness (ie, brain tumor, late stage syphilis), there is a clear physiologic pathway. This factor is not true for psychological factors interfering with a medical illness. The treatment of this diagnosis includes motivational interviewing, supportive or rehabilitative care, and the treatment of underlying or comorbid conditions, as well as patient education and engagement. A review of current medications with close attention to side effects can be often reveal the reason for poor compliance.

FACTITIOUS DISORDER

The classification of factitious disorder has not changed in the most recent DSM edition, except for the separation of "imposed on self" and "imposed on others" (previously referred to as Munchhausen syndrome).[1] Criteria include falsification of illness or injury, either physical or psychological. The patient presents as ill, injured, or impaired, but there is not necessarily an obvious gain for the behavior. Patients with factitious disorder show a similarity to patients with substance use or eating disorders in that they will attempt to conceal the behavior and its persistence.[1] Although some factitious disorder behaviors are criminal, such as causing a child illness or injury, factitious disorder criteria is the objective identification of deception and not the requirement of criminality.[1]

There may be clues in the presentation with behaviors "out of the norm," a lack of cooperation with the examination, and falsification of laboratory test results (ie, adding blood to the urine).[22] Physical examination may show self-harm with cutting, breaking bones, bruising, or causing a wound. Patients may take medications to simulate illness. Others may feign depression and suicidality owing to the death of family member or spouse when no death has occurred. Reports of bed sores on the elderly caused by a caregivers have been made. Patients have also falsified their medical records.

The diagnosis of this disorder may be difficult to identify because direct evidence of illness- or injury-inducing behaviors is needed. Patients suspected of this disorder may be hospitalized and often closed-circuit observation is needed to confirm the diagnosis. Some pediatric units have cameras in rooms to observe suspected caregiver behavior.[24] The diagnosis should specify single or recurrent episodes.[1]

The prevalence and etiology of factitious disorder are unclear; however, the disorders occur more frequently in those under age 40, female, and Caucasian and have a history of trauma, grief and/or health care experience. Other risk factors include family dysfunction to include enmeshment, separation, abuse, or conflict. Factitious disorder is found concurrently in patients with a history of mental illness (self or family), substance abuse, an extreme number of allergies, pain, and gastrointestinal, neurologic, and/or infectious disease.[10,22]

Although the management of factitious disorder generally should ensure the safety of the patient and family and close follow-up of a collaborative team, the prognosis is poor. It is important for clinicians to recall common risks and characteristics to minimize unnecessary work-ups.[23] Ethically we are obligated to report factitious disorder imposed on another person; however, the process is often avoided or passed on to the social work and protective service professionals. It is difficult, but the diagnosis should be presented to the patient by the team. Diagnosis and the documentation of risks and findings should be clear, as well as the long-term effects on outcomes and costs.[24,25] Psychiatric or psychological referral is needed; psychodynamic and eye movement desensitization and reprocessing therapy may be needed to address psychopathological and attachment deficits resulting from early trauma. Behavioral contracts aimed at reducing self-harm and the overuse of the medical system are often treated with CBT. As always, comorbid conditions should be referred or treated to remission.[22,24]

UNSPECIFIED SOMATIC SYMPTOMS AND RELATED DISORDER

Within the DSM, "unspecified" is always available and is used when patients present with symptoms similar to somatic symptom disorder but do not quite meet criteria for any 1 disorder. It is more commonly used when there are unusual circumstances or a lack of information.

Malingering

Malingering was not included in DSM 5 somatic disorders chapter, but is listed in the chapter, "Other Conditions That May Be a Focus of Clinical Attention," often referred to the V codes, under nonadherence.[1] Malingering is defined as purposefully falsifying or exaggerating symptoms for external incentives or secondary gain. The primary diagnosis is listed with an added diagnosis of malingering after the primary diagnosis.[1] For example, a primary diagnosis of a nonpressure ulcer of thigh (ICD 909) followed by malingering (ICD Z76.5 or DSM V65.2) to describe a patient transferred from local jail to ED who admitted to wanting to leave the jail owing to anxiety and self-inflicting the wound trying to resemble a spider bite he had in past. The diagnosis of malingering is seen more often in the military, correctional, or legal systems or insurance claims. When the patient fits the criteria for a somatic disorder, this code should not be used, even when the clinician thinks there may be intention. The traditional treatment strategy varies from confrontation to ignoring the intent and providing treatment. However, recognizing malingering as an indication of underlying need and pursuing this in a nonconfrontational, open conversation is usually more helpful.[1]

SUMMARY

The somatic disorders can be difficult to identify and manage. The goal is to improve function. The patient's symptoms can be exaggerated, dramatic and even misguided. Start with the Hippocratic oath "first, do no harm," take time to listen and acknowledge, and resist overevaluation in lieu of frequent follow-up. Somatic symptom disorder requires the presence of somatic symptoms and excessive thoughts regarding them. Illness anxiety disorder involves a fear of having or developing a disorder. Adjustment disorder will show a clear relationship to an identifiable stressor. Conversion disorder (functional neurologic symptom disorder) presents with the loss of motor or neurologic function without a physiologic basis. Factitious disorder presents with self-harm or harm to others. Increasing access with more frequent visits, screening for development of depression, especially in the elderly, may be needed. A focus on education and self-care should be encouraged.

Foundational to any definition of neuropsychiatry is the indelible inseparability of brain and thought, of mind and body, and of mental and physical.
—Stuart C. Yudofsky and Robert E. Hales[26]

CLINICS CARE POINTS

- If you hold negative feelings about patients in this illness category, work to change your paradigm.
- Validate and acknowledge patient symptoms and distress/dysfunction.
- Use empathy but maintain boundaries.
- Use frequent, time-limited appointments, which can decrease as function improves.
- Encourage CBT or counseling.
- Collaborate and coordinate with other providers.
- Your goal should be to increase function.
- Treatment can decrease symptoms, but is unlikely to remove them.
- Having 1 primary provider decreases doctor shopping and unnecessary costs.
- Use the CARE MD approach.
- Avoid the use of psychotropics if possible; it is advisable to focus medications on decreasing anxiety.
- Avoid the use of antipsychotics.
- Minimize health care costs through conservative management and encourage this in contacts with other providers who may be treating the patient.
- It is challenging, do not give up.

DISCLOSURE

Nothing to disclose.

REFERENCES

1. American Psychiatric Association. Diagnostic and statistical manual of mental disorders. 5th edition. Arlington, (VA): American Psychiatric Association; 2013.
2. Crocq MA. A history of anxiety: from Hippocrates to DSM. Dialogues Clin Neurosci 2015;17(3):319–25.
3. Black DW, Andreason NC. Introductory textbook of psychiatry. 6th edition. Arlington, (VA): American Psychiatric Publishing; 2014.
4. McCarron RM. Somatization in the primary care setting. Psychiatric Times; 2006. Available at: https://www.psychiatrictimes.com/view/somatization-primary-care-setting. Accessed July 20, 2020.
5. Kurlansik SL, Mafeei MS. Somatic symptom disorder. Am Fam Physician 2016; 93(1):49–54.
6. American Psychiatric Association. American Psychiatric Association: diagnostic and statistical manual of mental disorders. 3rd edition. Arlington, (VA): American Psychiatric Association; 1980.
7. American Psychiatric Association. Diagnostic and statistical manual of mental disorders. Fourth edition. Revised, Arlington, VA: American Association; 1994.
8. Crocq MA. The history of generalized anxiety disorder as a diagnostic category. Dialogues Clin Neurosci 2017;19(2):107–16.
9. Liu Y, Zhao J, Fan X, et al. Dysfunction in serotonergic and noradrenergic systems and somatic symptoms in psychiatric disorders. Front Psychiatry 2019; 10:286.

10. Bègue I, Adams C, Stone J, et al. Structural alterations in functional neurological disorder and related conditions: a software and hardware problem? Neuroimage Clin 2019;22:101798.
11. Shevlin M, Nolan E, Owczarek M, et al. COVID-19-related anxiety predicts somatic symptoms in the UK population [published online ahead of print, 2020 May 27]. Br J Health Psychol 2020. https://doi.org/10.1111/bjhp.12430.
12. Hawryluck L, Gold WL, Robinson S, et al. SARS control and psychological effects of quarantine, Toronto, Canada. Emerg Infect Dis 2004;10(7):1206–12.
13. Maples-Keller JL, Bunnell BE, Kim SJ, et al. The use of virtual reality technology in the treatment of anxiety and other psychiatric disorders. Harv Rev Psychiatry 2017;25(3):103–13.
14. Katon W, Ries RK, Kleinman A. The prevalence of somatization in primary care. Compr Psychiatry 1984;25(2):208–15.
15. Lakhan SE, Schofield KL. Mindfulness-based therapies in the treatment of somatization disorders: a systematic review and meta-analysis. PLoS One 2013;8(8): e71834.
16. Fallon BA, Liebowitz MR, Salmán E, et al. Fluoxetine for hypochondriacal patients without major depression. J Clin Psychopharmacol 1993;13(6):438–41.
17. Katzman MA, Bleau P, Blier P, et al. Canadian clinical practice guidelines for the management of anxiety, posttraumatic stress, and obsessive-compulsive disorders. BMC Psychiatry 2014;14(Suppl 1):S1.
18. Müller T, Mannel M, Murck H, et al. Treatment of somatoform disorders with St. John's wort: a randomized, double-blind, and placebo-controlled trial. Psychosom Med 2004;66(4):538–47.
19. Puzantian T, Carlat D. The medication fact book for psychiatric practice. 5th edition. Newburyport, (MA): Carlat Publishing; 2020.
20. Scarella TM, Boland RJ, Barsky AJ. Illness anxiety disorder: psychopathology, epidemiology, clinical characteristics, and treatment. Psychosom Med 2019; 81(5):398–407.
21. Anderson JR, Nakhate V, Stephen CD, et al. Functional (Psychogenic) neurological disorders: assessment and acute management in the emergency department. Semin Neurol 2019;39(1):102–14.
22. Banerjee A. Factitious disorders presenting as acute emergencies. Postgrad Med J 1994;70(820):68–73.
23. O'Connell N, Nicholson TR, Wessely S, et al. Characteristics of patients with motor functional neurological disorder in a large UK mental health service: a case-control study. Psychol Med 2020;50(3):446–55.
24. Tozzo P, Picozzi M, Caenazzo L. Munchausen Syndrome by Proxy: balancing ethical and clinical challenges for healthcare professionals Ethical consideration in factitious disorders. Clin Ter 2018;169(3):e129–34.
25. Gerstenblith TA, Stern TA. Primary care and consultation-liaison interventions for somatic symptom and related disorders. In: Gobbard GO, editor. Gabbard's treatments of psychiatric disorders. 5th edition. Washington, DC: 2014. p. 571–82.
26. Yudofsky SC, Hales RE. The indelible inseparability of brain and thought, of mind and body 2004. Available at: https://www.psychiatrictimes.com/view/indelible-inseparability-brain-and-thought-mind-and-body. Accessed August 2, 2020.

Something's Different
Recognizing Dementia and Delirium in the Hospital

Melissa Rodzen, PA-C[a],*, Lisa Tannenbaum, PA-C[b,c]

KEYWORDS

- Acute mental status change • Delirium • Dementia • Acute psychosis
- Alcohol withdrawal • Differential diagnosis

KEY POINTS

- Delirium may be the only indication of an emerging medical emergency and should be evaluated as such.
- Delirium is a very wide and diverse topic, resulting from a long list of differential diagnoses.
- Differentiating delirium, dementia, and psychiatric symptoms can be challenging.

INTRODUCTION

Mr Smith is a 75-year-old man with a history of alcoholism, type 2 diabetes, asthma, dementia, and bipolar disease admitted to the hospital for respiratory failure caused by coronavirus disease 2019 (COVID-19). He was successfully weaned off the ventilator this morning on day 5 of his hospital stay. Overnight, a nurse expressed concern regarding Mr Smith's behavior and mental status. When prompted for more detail, she stated, "Something's different" and requested a bedside evaluation.

In cases such as this, inpatient care teams are faced with a wide array of possible causes for altered mental status (AMS). Problems to consider include underlying dementia, psychiatric disorder, substance abuse or withdrawal, or any number of factors that can contribute to acute delirium. Identifying the correct cause of AMS in a timely manner can directly affect a patient's immediate treatment, overall hospital course, and long-term well-being.

[a] NYU Langone Emergency Department, 150 55th Street, Brooklyn, NY 11220, USA; [b] Victory Recovery Partners (VRP), Massapequa, NY, USA; [c] Bel Air Center for Addictions, 1202 Brighton Lane, Bel Air, MD 21014, USA
* Corresponding author.
E-mail address: melissa.rodzen@nyulangone.org

Physician Assist Clin 6 (2021) 527–540
https://doi.org/10.1016/j.cpha.2021.02.012
2405-7991/21/© 2021 Elsevier Inc. All rights reserved.

physicianassistant.theclinics.com

KNOWING THE DIFFERENTIAL

Diagnosing the precise cause of AMS in a hospitalized patient can be difficult for providers. Depending on the cause and duration of symptoms, it may be overlooked entirely without a high degree of suspicion and some knowledge of the patient's history, hospital course, and condition. It is a dangerous pitfall to assume that some level of alteration is present at baseline, especially for sick or elderly patients, when this may not be the case. Although the differential for AMS can be expansive, this article focuses on differentiating delirium, dementia, and psychiatric causes commonly observed in hospitalized patients such as the one described in the case earlier (**Fig 1**).

DEMENTIA

Dementia poses a significant burden to Americans and the health care system. In 2012, an estimated 8.8% of the population more than 65 years of age had some form of dementia. An increase in comorbidities along with a longer lifespan contribute to this higher incidence of dementia.[1] However, despite this high prevalence, many misconceptions still exist among clinicians when treating patients with confirmed or suspected dementia. Often, dementia is used as an umbrella term in medical settings to explain a patient's AMS, and it can range from mild forgetfulness to frank hallucinations and loss of orientation. However, acute changes of cognition or attention may be overlooked without a firm understanding of dementia, its causes, and typical progression. By definition, dementia is not a disease entity within itself but is a broad term

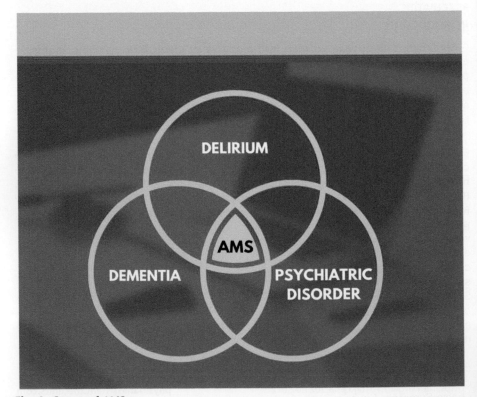

Fig. 1. Causes of AMS.

used to describe cognitive decline. This decline may be caused by a wide range of distinct diseases or even a combination of disease processes simultaneously (**Table 1**).

Although many patients similar to the index patient enter the hospital with an existing diagnosis of dementia, it is also useful to be familiar with disease risk factors as well as the broad diagnostic criteria for dementia. Dementia is now referred to as major neurocognitive disorder, as described by The Diagnostic and Statistical Manual of Mental Disorders, Fifth Edition (DSM-5).[4] Knowledge of disease risk factors and diagnostic criteria may prove useful for patients who show signs or symptoms without having had a formal diagnosis (**Box 1**).

A WORD ON SUNDOWNING

Colloquially, the term sundowning is used to describe increased agitation, confusion, behavioral disturbance, or disorientation during evening hours in patients with dementia. The term is used as a description of behavior and is not inherently a diagnosis.[5] Although the phenomenon has been observed for decades, there is a lack of formal acknowledgment from major medical bodies and it is not mentioned in the DSM-5. As such, it remains poorly defined, insufficiently studied, and overwhelmingly abstract. Without clear differentiation between sundowning and delirium, clinicians should remain wary of any acute AMS changes and maintain high clinical suspicion for alternative disorders when appropriate.[6]

PSYCHIATRIC DISORDERS

AMS changes may also be a result of psychiatric disorders, and these should be considered even when symptoms have previously been well controlled. Changes in environment, routine, medications, or an acute illness may exacerbate symptoms of psychiatric illness, resulting in behavioral changes, delirium, pseudodementia, or even frank psychosis. While evaluating a patient with a known psychiatric illness, skilled clinicians consider the individual patient's history and symptoms to differentiate between exacerbation of a chronic illness and development of a possible new disease.

PSYCHOTIC PATIENTS

Psychotic disorders and their definitions have undergone substantial changes in recent years. Although psychotic episodes were at one time associated almost exclusively with schizophrenia, the DSM-5 has reclassified psychotic disorders and schizophrenia to include a spectrum of psychological processes.[4] While evaluating a patient with hallucinations or delusions, it is important to remember that, although their presence is central to diagnosing psychosis, not all delusions or hallucinations are psychotic. When an individual maintains insight, for example, stating, "I see a giant spider on the wall, but I know it is not really there," the hallucination is not psychotic. Such symptoms are psychotic when the individual cannot distinguish the hallucination or delusion from reality. It is also essential to distinguish true hallucinations from illusions, especially in elderly patients who may have visual or hearing impairments (**Box 2**).

In order to create a more structured diagnosis and evaluation of patients with psychosis, the American Psychiatric Association has released an 8-item survey to assist clinicians in measuring psychosis severity.[4] The Clinician-rated Dimensions of Psychosis Symptom Severity Scale measures the presence or absence of the following

Table 1
Common diseases associated with dementia

Type	Onset	Identifying Features	Typical Progression
Alzheimer dementia	Increasing incidence after age 65 y[2]	• The most common type of dementia accounting for up to 60% of all cases[1] • Early anterograde amnesia • Associated with amyloid plaques and tau neurofibrillary tangles in brain[2] • Associated with apolipoprotein E polymorphism[2]	Gradual progression over years[2]
Parkinson dementia	Several years after onset of Parkinson disease	• Occurs in up to 30% of patients with Parkinson disease • Should only be diagnosed in patients with known, well-established Parkinson disease • Fluctuations of attention and onset of hallucinations in late disease	Gradual progression years after Parkinson disease symptom onset[2]
Lewy Body dementia	Typical onset after age 50 y	• Neurocognitive dysfunction precedes or occurs within 1 y of parkinsonism[3] • Motor symptoms minimally responsive to carbidopa/levodopa[3] • Often associated with visual hallucinations early in disease • Neuroleptics often exacerbate symptoms[3] • Fluctuations in attention, behaviors, personality, and alertness[3]	Variable progression with fluctuations in attention, behavior, personality, and memory Overall decline over years[3]
Frontotemporal dementia	Age 35–75y Onset rare after age 75 y	• Symptoms primarily in language deficits, behavior changes, and personality changes[2] • Memory loss less pervasive than executive function dysfunction in early stages	Gradual decline over years[2]

(continued on next page)

Table 1 (continued)			
Type	Onset	Identifying Features	Typical Progression
Vascular dementia	Rare before age 65 y	• May be the result of ischemic, hemorrhagic, anoxic, or hypoxic brain damage • Often is accompanied by a history of hypertension and atherosclerosis[2]	Gradual but stepwise decline[2]

Data from Hugo J, Ganguli M. Dementia and cognitive impairment: epidemiology, diagnosis, and treatment and Gomperts SN. Lewy Body Dementias: Dementia With Lewy Bodies and Parkinson Disease Dementia. Continuum (Minneap Minn).

over the previous 7 days on an ongoing basis to monitor improvements or worsening of psychosis[4]:

- Hallucinations
- Delusions
- Disorganized speech
- Abnormal psychomotor behavior

Box 1
Dementia risk factors

- Polypharmacy
- Increasing age
- Female sex
- Lower education level
- Genetic factors
  ○ Apolipoprotein E polymorphism
- Chronic comorbidities
  ○ Hypertension
  ○ Hyperlipidemia
  ○ Coronary artery disease
  ○ Diabetes mellitus
  ○ Tobacco abuse[a]
  ○ Heavy alcohol abuse
  ○ Obesity
  ○ Obstructive sleep apnea
  ○ Depression
  ○ Posttraumatic stress disorder
- Traumatic brain injury
- History of stroke

[a] Smoking is associated with increased risk for all forms of dementia except Parkinson disease, for which it is consistently observed to be protective. This finding is possibly caused by nicotine effects on cholinergic receptors.

Data from Gomperts SN. Lewy Body Dementias: Dementia With Lewy Bodies and Parkinson Disease Dementia. Continuum (Minneap Minn).

Box 2
Hallucinations, illusions, and delusions

Important definitions

- Hallucination: perceived sense (visual, auditory, tactile) without the presence of external stimulus
  - For example: seeing a tiger that is not present in the room

- Illusion: misperceiving an external stimulus that is actually present
  - For example: mistaking a chair in the room for a tiger

- Delusion: a fixed, false belief that persists despite proof of the contrary
  - For example: believing a tiger ate the nurse despite being shown the nurse alive and uninjured

Data from Arciniegas DB. Psychosis. Continuum (Minneap Minn). 2015;21(3 Behavioral Neurology and Neuropsychiatry).[7]

- Negative symptoms
- Impaired cognition
- Depression
- Mania

When a patient presents with psychotic symptoms, the importance of a thorough history and collateral information from those familiar with the patient cannot be overestimated. Historical information is essential for differentiating new-onset psychosis versus recurrent psychosis in those with known psychiatric disorder. Clinicians should also be familiar with the psychiatric disorders and patterns likely to cause a disconnect with reality, which include schizotypal personality disorder, schizophreniform disorder, schizophrenia disorder, schizoaffective disorder, delusional disorder, brief psychotic disorder, bipolar disease with psychotic features, and major depressive disorder with psychotic features.[7]

MOODY PATIENTS

Mood disorders are less commonly the source of AMS in the inpatient setting, with the following exceptions:

- Pseudodementia: depressive states cause decreased cognition, which can sometimes be severe enough to mimic dementia. It can be difficult to differentiate dementia from depression in older populations. It is also possible for the two to coexist. Depression in the elderly should be noted and addressed to prevent diagnostic confusion while evaluating cognitive deficits. Recent data suggest there may be a role for neurocognitive tests when attempting to differentiate dementia and reversible cognitive deficits caused by depression.[8]
- Bipolar disease: mania or depressive episodes sometimes include psychotic features. When differentiating symptoms of bipolar disease from other conditions, timing may be a key feature. Symptoms of mania must occur for a period of 1 week or more for diagnosis; symptoms of hypomania must occur for a period of 4 days or more for diagnosis; symptoms of depression must last 2 weeks.[4]
  - One to 2 episodes (mania plus depression) per year is typical of bipolar disease with asymptomatic periods between episodes.
  - A word on rapid cycling: this term is not used to describe mood swings over minutes, hours, or even days in most cases. Rapid cycling is not a diagnosis

or type of bipolar disease. It describes an individual with bipolar disease who experiences 4 or more distinct episodes over the course of 1 1year.[4]
- Borderline personality disorder: although not a mood disorder, borderline personality disorder is commonly associated with abrupt changes in behavior and mood lability.

INTOXICATED OR WITHDRAWING PATIENTS

Changes in mental status may be caused by acute intoxication or withdrawal. A reported or suspected history of substance abuse, or particularly heavy or frequent alcohol use, should increase the index of suspicion for withdrawal as a cause of AMS. Identifying at-risk patients and recognizing signs of withdrawal before progression may significantly reduce the number of patients who have either AMS or delirium tremens (DTs).

In patients dependent on alcohol, withdrawal symptoms may begin as soon as 8 hours after decrease of blood alcohol levels. Notably, alcohol withdrawal syndrome does not begin with cognitive symptoms but with autonomic hyperactivity such as increased heart rate and blood pressure, nausea, vomiting, headache, tremors, sweating, and/or anxiety. Although anxiety may become severe, there is no clouding of sensorium unless withdrawal is allowed to progress. When left untreated, withdrawal symptoms typically peak around 72 hours from initial withdrawal from alcohol and progress to psychomotor agitation, visual, auditory and/or tactile hallucinations, and eventually seizures or even death.[9] True DTs occurs only if the withdrawal is not treated at any previous stage and results in true delirium.

Benzodiazepines are inhibitory drugs with mechanisms of action similar to those of alcohol. As such, withdrawal from benzodiazepines may cause similar symptoms to alcohol withdrawal, including progression to seizures and delirium if left untreated. Severe withdrawal usually occurs within 4 days of abrupt cessation of the patient taking high doses of medication daily.[10]

In the hospital setting, acute intoxication with illicit substances is common. Any suspicion of acute intoxication should be investigated despite inpatient status.

DELIRIUM

Similar to dementia, delirium is an umbrella diagnosis. The term delirium originated more than 1000 years ago and its definition has evolved over time. The term is now used to describe acute fluctuations to attention, awareness, or orientation caused by any medical condition. It is often reversible and sometimes unpredictable, posing a diagnostic challenge to many clinicians. The onset of delirium is often precipitated by modifiable influences on preexisting chronic risks (eg, infection in a patient with Alzheimer disease). Because risk factors play such a significant role in the development of delirium, utmost care should be taken to minimize modifiable risks in the inpatient setting, especially for elderly patients with some form of dementia (**Box 3**).

Fluctuating deficits to attention, cognition, awareness, and orientation are characteristic of delirium. These deficits may be cause for admission or may have an abrupt onset during a patient's hospital stay. However, delirium frequently remains unrecognized in the inpatient setting. When it is recognized, it is most often in an acutely agitated, hallucinating patient. However, hyperactive delirium is only 1 of 3 presentations. Delirium may also present with negative symptoms such as lethargy, decreased responsiveness to interviews, decreased purposeful movement, and/or decreased engagement with surroundings. This hypoactive delirium may be misdiagnosed as

---

Box 3
Delirium risk factors

- Hearing or vision impairment
- Immobilization
- Medications and polypharmacy
- Acute neurologic disease
- Metabolic derangement
- Recent surgery
- Admission to the intensive care unit
- Pain
- Anxiety, depression
- Sleep deprivation
- Age>65 y
- Male sex
- Cognitive impairment
- Multiple comorbidities

Data from Fong TG, Tulebaev SR, Inouye SK. Delirium in elderly adults: diagnosis, prevention and treatment. Nat Rev Neurol. 2009.[11]

---

depression or dementia, especially in elderly populations. A detailed history of a patient's baseline mentation and behavior can help prevent such errors.[11]

Although the identification of delirium alone may prove challenging to many providers, it is only half of the answer. By definition, delirium must be directly related to a physiologic cause. Once suspected, further investigations must be pursued to identify the cause (**Fig. 2**). Finding the underlying cause of delirium is essential to reversing changes in mental status and restoring patients to baseline mentation.

THE HISTORY

The evaluation of AMS begins with a thorough history and medication review. Without gathering this information, the cause for AMS is nearly impossible to diagnose correctly in a timely manner (**Table 2**). Considering details of symptoms (onset, timing,

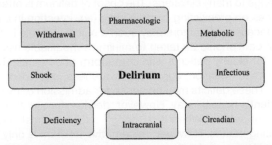

Fig. 2. Causes of delirium. (*Data from* Huang J, By, Huang J, Last full review/revision Dec 2019| Content last modified Dec 2019. Delirium - Neurologic Disorders. Merck Manuals Professional Edition.[12])

Table 2 History considerations	
Additional Questions	**Considerations**
Was there any possible inciting event around the time of symptom onset?	• Fall • Medication administration • Cessation of substance • Change in environment • Recent procedure • Sleep deprivation[13]
What are the specific symptoms?	• Deficits to cognition • Deficits to attention • Disorientation • Agitation • Lethargy • Psychosis[13]
What is the progression and status of symptoms?	• Abrupt onset • Gradual onset • Constant symptoms • Fluctuating symptoms • Worsening • Improving[13]
Associated signs or symptoms?	• Palpitations • Nausea, vomiting, diarrhea • Vision changes • Dizziness • Pain • Anxiety • Depression[13]
Risk factors?	• Age • Medical history • Surgical history • Social history • Psychiatric history • Recent procedures • Medications and polypharmacy • History of similar symptoms[13]

Data from European Delirium Association; American Delirium Society. The DSM-5 criteria, level of arousal and delirium diagnosis: inclusiveness is safer. BMC Med. 2014.

character, severity, duration, order) or modifying factors can direct clinicians toward a cause. The importance of medical, psychiatric, surgical, medication, social, and family history, with special attention to risk factors, cannot be overlooked.

THE OBJECTIVE EXAMINATION

The Case

An hour into your shift, you receive the call from the nurse stating there was something different about Mr Smith's behavior. With additional probing, you learn that, although he was at his baseline during rounds 1 hour ago, he called for his nurse soon after, asking when they would be docking the ship. He also refused to ambulate to the restroom in fear of sharks in the water surrounding his bed. The nurse denies the possibility of falls or trauma and states that, other than anxiety, the patient denies any complaints. He did not miss any doses of medications, nor did he begin anything new. On further chart review, you learn Mr Smith's dementia is caused by early-stage Alzheimer disease. His bipolar disease has been well controlled on lithium for many years and he has not required admission because of psychiatric illness since his youth. Although he experiences occasional relapses, his alcohol use has been controlled for years as well. His diabetes is managed with insulin. His laboratory tests and chest radiograph this morning were unremarkable.

The Examination

A full physical examination should be completed when possible but may be difficult because of patient cooperation or ability. However, a limited examination can still provide vital information, especially when the patient is unable to communicate effectively. Even in patients with chronic mentation deficits, acute changes should be fully evaluated and emergent or reversible causes should be excluded before being attributed to exacerbation or delirium caused by chronic conditions. Be wary if physical examination findings are incongruent with initial impressions. For example, the presence of abnormal vital signs and lack of orientation in a patient initially assumed to be depressed. Other pitfalls to avoid are mistaking language barriers, chronic hearing or visual deficits, or residual changes from prior stroke or injury for acute changes during evaluation.

The Case

A focused physical examination of Mr Smith is performed, revealing mild tachypnea to a rate of 23 breaths/min with normal oxygen saturation on 2-L nasal cannula. He is afebrile with a heart rate of 80 beats/min and blood pressure of 140/85 mm Hg. He is disoriented to time, place, and situation, but otherwise is without neurologic deficits. He has obvious psychomotor agitation and anxiety, and frequently tries to remove his nasal cannula to "get off the boat" during his examination, requiring redirection. The rest of the physical examination is unremarkable and per his baseline. He has no signs of trauma.

The Laboratory Tests

Because AMS can have multiple causes, laboratory and imaging evaluation should be guided by findings from the history and physical examination. Blood glucose should be checked at the bedside during initial evaluation to address severe hyperglycemia or hypoglycemia. A complete blood panel and chemistry are warranted to evaluate common potential causes of confusion, including signs of dehydration, electrolyte imbalance, kidney or liver abnormalities, anemia, and/or infections (including sexually transmitted infections). Urinalysis is often abnormal, especially in the elderly. Blood gas and lactate may support a diagnosis of sepsis, acidosis, or alkalosis. Cardiac enzymes are also reasonable in patients unable to provide history or report symptoms.

When history and physical examination lend suspicion, ammonia levels, thyroid function, toxicology, alcohol levels, and other substance or medication levels may be indicated. Creatinine kinase levels are often increased in postictal patients. Thiamine and B_{12} levels should be considered in patients with chronic alcoholism or malnutrition, or may be medication induced. Blood cultures may also be considered even in the absence of fever if concerns for infection are present.

Although autoimmune diseases such as lupus have been associated with encephalopathies, laboratory evaluation in an acute setting is unlikely to yield diagnostic results, and many inflammatory markers are nonspecific. Similarly, free cortisol levels are unlikely to yield a definitive diagnosis at the exact time of symptom onset. However, if suspicion is high or if another cause is not identified through evaluation, lumbar puncture should be considered with attention to opening pressure during the procedure. If evaluation remains negative, other causes, such as syphilis, listeria, human immunodeficiency virus, or tick-borne illness, should be considered.

The Case

After comparing Mr Smith's current condition with his baseline, you recognize an acute change in mental status and initiate a work-up starting with laboratory evaluation. This evaluation reveals a mild leukocytosis, an acute kidney injury, and mild respiratory acidosis, which is improved from the time of extubation. His urinalysis, ammonia, thyroid function, cardiac enzymes, thiamine, B_{12}, and alcohol levels are all within normal limits.

The Images

Most AMS work-ups include a chest radiograph because it is low risk, portable, and inexpensive, and may reveal several disorders. Neuroimaging infrequently yields diagnosis when obvious signs of stroke are not present. When signs of infection, dehydration, or history of dementia present, risk of focal lesion on neuroimaging in delirium has been found to be as low as 2%.[11] If there is any concern for intracranial disorder or if a lumbar puncture is going to be performed, a computed tomography (CT) brain should be completed. If work-up does not reveal a cause, further evaluation of the brain with MRI and electroencephalogram should be considered. If acutely abnormal or sudden vital sign or hemoglobin changes are noted, aortic dissection or retroperitoneal bleed should be suspected and followed up with the appropriate imaging.

The Case

Concerned about Mr Smith's mental status change, a chest radiograph and electrocardiogram (ECG) are performed. His chest radiograph shows patchy opacities improved compared with earlier, which is consistent with his COVID-19 course. His ECG remains normal sinus rhythm without acute changes. Because Mr Smith does not have any focal neurologic deficits, a CT brain is deferred at this time. Mr Smith lacks meningeal signs or high suspicion for infection based on his laboratory results, so a lumbar puncture is also not completed pending further work-up.

TYING IT ALL TOGETHER

Delirium is a common but often unrecognized condition. It affects up to 24% of the hospitalized community and may occur in up to 87% of elderly patients who are admitted and treated in the intensive care unit (ICU).[11] Acute changes should be promptly evaluated and never assumed to be an exacerbation of chronic illness without a thorough history and evaluation to exclude delirium. Although psychiatric disease or dementia can cause changes in cognition or behavior, or even provoke delirium, they are diagnostically distinct. Psychiatric disease and dementia need to be differentiated from delirium when present. Any instances of delirium should be promptly evaluated as a medical emergency. Once a cause is identified, it should be managed and steps should be taken to prevent subsequent occurrences.

Despite the often reversible nature of acute delirium, there exists long-term consequences that further highlight the importance of prevention and identification of delirium. Patients who experience delirium while hospitalized have comparable mortalities at 1 year after discharge with those diagnosed with sepsis or myocardial infarct.[14] Even patients without dementia show long-term cognitive decline after experiencing a delirium episode in the ICU. Furthermore, longer duration of delirium is associated with worsening cognitive function over time.[15]

However, steps can be taken to limit the risk of delirium. In several studies, family involvement in care has been shown to decrease instances of delirium.[16] Eyeglasses or hearing aids can decrease confusion, and physical restraints should be avoided to prevent sensory impairment. Patients, especially those with dementia, should be frequently reoriented. Sleep interruptions should be avoided whenever possible. Pain control, laboratory abnormalities, nutrition, and hydration status should be reviewed daily.[16] Known risks of substance dependence or abuse should be reviewed and monitored for relapse or withdrawal symptoms. At-risk patients should be frequently monitored using the appropriate clinical scales for any concerns.

The Case

Mr Smith's case is reviewed with the team during morning rounds. Because of the rapid onset and fluctuating nature of his symptoms, he is suspected to have developed ICU delirium associated with COVID-19. In addition to the inherent risk for delirium associated with intensive care and severe illness, patients such as Mr Smith who are infected with coronavirus are also at an increased risk for delirium because of coronavirus itself. The virus has the ability to invade the central nervous system to directly cause neurologic symptoms. Some patients may even present with delirium before the development of fever or respiratory symptoms.[17]

The team decides to implement strategies to reduce instances of delirium in Mr Smith. He is provided with a tablet device to video communicate with his family while in isolation. He is also provided with ear plugs at night and is regularly reoriented during the day by nursing staff. The medical team reviews his medications to limit polypharmacy wherever possible. He continues to improve and is eventually discharged without further events.

SUMMARY

AMS is a common occurrence in hospital settings and carries a wide differential. Although AMS may be related to chronic disease (eg, dementia or psychiatric illness), a detailed history, medication review, physical examination, and laboratory and imaging evaluations are always indicated during unexplained acute changes. Changes in attention, behavior, and language in dementia depend on the type and severity of dementia but rarely present as abrupt changes. Although a hospitalization may make AMS obvious, with deeper questioning, the family may have noticed previous changes at home. Psychiatric illness and dementia are not frequently associated with changes in vital signs or laboratory abnormalities. Abrupt changes, especially changes in attention or orientation, should be evaluated as delirium. Reversible causes should be addressed and future instances should be avoided to prevent long-term cognitive decline and mortality.

Risk factors for delirium, including hearing and vision defects of older adults, should be minimized. Suspicion should not be limited to the elderly. Because of the frequency and long-term consequences of delirium, preventive measures should be taken in any hospitalized patient at risk. Any occurrence should be rapidly evaluated, diagnosed, and treated to alleviate AMS but also prevent long-term cognitive decline.

CLINICS CARE POINTS

- Altered mental status (AMS) can have a wide variety of potential causes, and correctly identifying them has huge implications for diagnosis, treatment, and ultimately patient outcomes even after they are discharged from an acute care setting.

- 'Dementia' is often used as an umbrella term to cover a variety of causes of cognitive impairment or decline, and careful consideration of patient's baseline should be made when determining if dementia is truly present in AMS.

- Acute physical illness may exacerbate or change the presentation of psychiatric illness and should be considered as contributing factors to AMS even when a chronic psychiatric illness is also present.

- In order to create a more structured diagnosis and evaluation of patients with psychosis, the American Psychiatric Association has released an 8-item survey to assist clinicians in measuring psychosis severity.

- Intoxication and withdrawal are also important contributing factors to AMS that should be considered in patients with appropriate risk factors.

DISCLOSURE

M. Rodzen, no disclosures; L. Tannenbaum, no disclosures.

REFERENCES

1. Fishman E. Risk of developing dementia at older ages in the United States. Demography 2017;54(5):1897–919.
2. Hugo J, Ganguli M. Dementia and cognitive impairment: epidemiology, diagnosis, and treatment. Clin Geriatr Med 2014;30(3):421–42.
3. Gomperts SN. Lewy body dementias: dementia with lewy bodies and parkinson disease dementia. Continuum (Minneap Minn) 2016;22(2 Dementia):435–63.
4. American Psychiatric Association. Diagnostic and statistical manual of mental disorders. Fifth edition. Arlington, VA: Author; 2013.
5. Bliwise DL. What is sundowning? J Am Geriatr Soc 1994;42(9):1009–11.
6. Canevelli M, Valletta M, Trebbastoni A, et al. Sundowning in dementia: clinical relevance, pathophysiological determinants, and therapeutic approaches. Frontiers; 2016. Available at: https://www.frontiersin.org/articles/10.3389/fmed.2016.00073/full. Accessed August 1, 2020.
7. Arciniegas DB. Psychosis. Continuum (Minneap Minn) 2015;21(3):715–36.
8. Kang H, Zhao F, You L, et al. Pseudo-dementia: a neuropsychological review. Ann Indian Acad Neurol 2014;17(2):147–54.
9. Schuckit M. Recognition and management of withdrawal delirium (delirium tremens). N Engl J Med 2014;371(22):2109–13.
10. Greenberg MI. Benzodiazepine withdrawal: potentially fatal, commonly missed following benzodiazepine cessation, withdrawal symptoms may begin within 24 hours or take up to two weeks to develop. Emerg Med News 2001;23(12):18.
11. Fong TG, Tulebaev SR, Inouye SK. Delirium in elderly adults: diagnosis, prevention and treatment. Nat Rev Neurol 2009;5(4):210–20.
12. Huang J. Last full review/revision Dec 2019| Content last modified Dec 2019. Delirium - neurologic disorders. Merck Manuals Professional Edition. Available at: https://www.merckmanuals.com/professional/neurologic-disorders/delirium-and-dementia/delirium#v1036383. Accessed July 27, 2020.
13. European Delirium Association, American Delirium Society. The DSM-5 criteria, level of arousal and delirium diagnosis: inclusiveness is safer. BMC Med 2014; 12:141.
14. Gross AL, Jones RN, Habtemariam DA, et al. Delirium and long-term cognitive trajectory among persons with dementia. Arch Intern Med 2012;172(17):1324–31.

15. van den Boogaard M, Schoonhoven L, Evers AW, et al. Delirium in critically ill patients: impact on long-term health-related quality of life and cognitive functioning. Crit Care Med 2012;40(1):112–8.
16. Martinez F, Tobar C, Hill N. Preventing delirium: should non-pharmacological, multicomponent interventions be used? A systematic review and meta-analysis of the literature. Age Ageing 2015;44(2):196–204.
17. Cipriani G, Danti S, Nuti A, et al. A complication of coronavirus disease 2019: delirium. Acta Neurol Belg 2020;120(4):927–32.

No Man Is an Island

Isolation and Mental Health in the Twenty-First Century

Michael Asbach, MPAS, PA-C

KEYWORDS

- Mental health • Technology • Artificial intelligence • Telepsychiatry • Loneliness
- Mhealth • Telehealth • Isolation

KEY POINTS

- The twenty-first century is experiencing an economic transformation driven by technology and automation.
- Society has become more individualistic, leading to more loneliness.
- Loneliness drives negative physical and emotional health outcomes.
- The future of mental health care includes innovations in psychopharmacology, changes to the care delivery model through telemedicine and mobile applications, and the adoption of artificial intelligence as a clinical support tool.

INTRODUCTION

Mental illness has plagued humans since the dawn of time. Authors have documented struggles with mental health in nearly every culture and society throughout history. Although descriptions of syndromes in ancient texts are vague and difficult to correlate to modern medicine, the presence of mental illness was well-documented. Ancient Mesopotamian texts described mental illness as a form of demon possession treated by priests.[1] Ancient Babylonian, Egyptian, and Indian cultures also believed that mental illness stemmed from the supernatural. In ancient Greece, opinions were divided whether mental illness was a spiritual or biologic affliction. Hippocrates, who is often considered the Father of Medicine, categorized mental illness as melancholia, mania, and phrenitis.[2] Hippocrates postulated that mental illness was due to an imbalance in the body's humors. Humors included yellow bile, black bile, phlegm, and blood. Bloodletting along with religious interventions were common treatments in Ancient Greek society.[2]

The Ancient Roman Empire brought along an evolution in the understanding and treatment of mental illness. The philosopher Cicero hypothesized that melancholia

DENT Neurologic Institute, 3980 Sheridan Drive, Suite 500, Amherst, NY 14226, USA
E-mail address: Asbach.mike@gmail.com

Physician Assist Clin 6 (2021) 541–553
https://doi.org/10.1016/j.cpha.2021.03.003
2405-7991/21/© 2021 Elsevier Inc. All rights reserved.
physicianassistant.theclinics.com

was caused by fear, grief, and other internal influences. This recording was one of the earliest suggesting that the source of depression was a psychological cause.[3] Greek and Roman society represented a significant evolution in attitudes toward mental illness. Both cultures identified disease influence alterations to the sensorium versus supernatural or divinely influenced changes in mentation. The advent of the Christian era did not eliminate the supernatural attributions of mental illness. Rather, Christianity shifted the psychological mysticism from pagan to monotheistic explanations. Like many other aspects of science and philosophy, the Dark Ages were a time of regression in societal attitudes and treatments of mental illness. The church often interpreted mental disorders as witchcraft. In 1484, Pope Innocent VIII declared Germany full of witches. Historians estimate that upwards of 50,000 people were killed under the guise of witch hunts. Common treatments of mental illness in Dark Ages included bloodletting and an involuntary treatment where the individual was hurled into the river to help them come to their senses.[4]

In 1844, a group of asylum superintendents formed a society that would later become the American Psychiatric Association.[5] Throughout the years, psychiatry has evolved and changed as new understandings of the brain developed, but also to fit the societal mental health needs as cultural norms changed. Mental illness has been present throughout human history, but the recognition, understanding, and treatment of these conditions is continually updated. Each generation and society has encountered different presentations of mental illness and has adopted different treatment approaches based on cultural beliefs and norms. The twenty-first century has been an era defined by transformational change in how humans live, work, and interact. Mental illness and treatments have also changed in the twenty-first century.

TWENTY-FIRST CENTURY PROBLEMS: ECONOMIC DISRUPTION

In history, there have been periods of rapid social disruption and transformation. For thousands of years, people resided in a single community. They would live and work in a small town or village, possibly not ever traveling more than a few dozen miles from their birthplace throughout their lives. The Industrial Revolution shifted Western societies from an agrarian to an industrial economy. This disruption, driven by technological change, led to new economic opportunities. Rapid change also brought displacement as some people struggled to adapt to the new economy. People were pushed from small towns and farms into large industrial cities in pursuit of a better life, but they often found harsh conditions and less community support. The disruptions of the early twentieth century created new social problems and ailments. Prohibition was initially enacted with broad social support in an effort to address an unintended consequence of urbanization. The Industrial Revolution also led to widening inequality, which contributed to social upheaval.[6]

Presently, a similar type of cultural shift is occurring, starting with the advent of the information age and progressing toward widespread adoption of artificial intelligence. As of May 2019, the most common jobs in America were retail salespersons, fast food and counter workers, and cashiers.[7] Experts estimate that approximately 50% of current work activities are automatable with currently available technologies. By 2030, up to 14% of the global workforce may need to change their occupational category in response to this technological disruption.[8] The transition to automation was already occurring before the global novel coronavirus disease 2019 (COVID-19) pandemic. The global crisis will likely accelerate the adoption of automation as firms seek investments to maintain operations while limiting human interaction, along with the lower borrowing costs designed to stimulate business investment.[9]

In addition to job loss secondary to technological advances, work in industries that are insulated from automation are experiencing psychosocial disruption. Before the COVID-19 pandemic, telework was being adopted, but more slowly than predicted.[10] The pandemic is now forcing business investment into remote technology that will likely persist beyond the current crisis. Telework carries benefits and drawbacks for employees. Workers report a better quality of life and a more satisfying work–life balance. However, telework can also lead to personal and professional isolation. For many Americans, work is a primary source of identity and community.[11] At this time, it remains unclear what effects long-term or permanent telework may have on workers' physical and emotional well-being.

Unemployment and mental health struggles do seem to have a causal relationship.[12,13] As early as the Great Depression, psychologists have argued that involuntary joblessness leads to anxiety, self-doubt, and a sense of helplessness.[14] Research also suggests that the psychosocial quality of work determines whether employment has mental health benefits.[15] The importance of work as a source of structure, stability, and purpose makes the current trends of economic disruption ominous. Opioid abuse has steadily increased in the past 2 decades and has heavily impacted rural Appalachia. Research has identified that rates of opioid misuse are persistently higher in coal mining regions of Appalachia compared with noncoal mining Appalachian communities.[16] The decline of coal as a viable energy source has devastated entire regions of the country, leading to socioeconomic decimation. The economic disruptions of automation, outsourcing, and artificial intelligence will only accelerate these seismic changes to communities, leading to great mental health struggles.

TWENTY-FIRST CENTURY PROBLEMS: LONELINESS

On July 13, 1995, Chicago experienced some of the most extreme temperatures in recorded history. The recorded temperature at Chicago Midway Airport reached 106°F and the heat index was an astounding 126°F.[17] Chicago is not a city that is accustomed to extreme heat and many poor urban residents lacked access to air conditioning, and those who did ran their units to the point of power grid collapse in many parts of the city. By September 1995, researchers attributed 739 deaths to the heatwave.[17] Groups that suffered higher fatality rates included the elderly, poor, the sick, and those who lacked access to transportation. Researcher Eric Klinenberg identified a trend in the fatality data; those with cohesive social contacts fared better than those who were isolated and alone.[18]

Several urban, poor, and predominantly minority communities fared far better than communities of similar socioeconomic status. For example, Latinos accounted for 25% of the city population but only 2% of the heat wave fatalities, despite a disproportionately low socioeconomic status. Klinenberg[18] concluded that social relationships and communities were protective factors, whereas high death tolls were observed in areas of the city that had been abandoned by most residents, leaving the unconnected and isolated. Elderly or at-risk residents who lived in communities with strong cohesive bonds fared better because people checked in on them and ensured they were safe. The Chicago heat wave can be viewed as a social disaster rather than a natural one. The death toll was heavily influenced by deficits in Chicago's social environment that contributed to a population of isolated individuals who lived and died alone.

Loneliness is a growing epidemic in America. Although loneliness can be difficult to define or measure, there is consensus that isolation is detrimental to overall health. A meta-analysis concluded that objective and subjective social isolation corresponded with a 26% to 32% increase in mortality.[19] This increase in mortality has been compared with smoking 15 cigarettes per day.[20] Loneliness is linked to many health problems, including depression, anxiety, self-harm, substance abuse, heart disease, and dementia.[21] Diseases of despair, often defined as suicide or drug- and alcohol-related deaths, have steadily increased in the past few decades. Life expectancy for White Americans aged 45 to 54 is declining owing to the increase in premature deaths.[22]

In the past 50 years, the share of American households with just 1 person has increased from 17% to 28%. The rate of marriage in the United States has decreased by approximately 20% in the past 2 decades.[23] This finding is particularly concerning for men, who are at an increased risk of loneliness and isolation because men tend to stop expanding their friendships by their early 30s. This situation makes bachelors susceptible to loneliness. In men, social connection is driven by their spouses and children. A recent British YouGov poll found that nearly one-fifth of men report having no close friends and 32% had no one they counted as a best friend.[24] In the 1995 Chicago heat wave, there were 4 times more fatalities among men than among women.[25]

Although many people already struggled with loneliness, the COVID-19 pandemic has exacerbated this crisis. Surveys conducted in April 2020 by SocialPro and ValuePenguin reported that 30% to 47% of American adults felt lonelier than usual.[26,27] SocialPro found that 34% of millennials reported feeling lonely always or often owing to the pandemic.[26] Even before the COVID-19 pandemic, rates of loneliness were significantly higher in younger generations. In a 2019 survey released by health insurer Cigna, more than 70% Millennials and Generation Z reported being lonely. Baby Boomers and the Greatest Generation reported loneliness in 50% and 38% of respondents, respectively.[28] The increase of loneliness in younger generations is a concerning statistical. This trend supports the theory that a cultural shift is occurring leaving people without deep and meaningful social connections. This circumstance will continue to have broad implications on mental health through the next few decades as economic disruption and cultural norms continue to move toward more individualized activities.

TWENTY-FIRST CENTURY PROBLEMS: SOCIAL CAPITAL

Harvard social scientist Robert Putnam has been researching how Americans live and interact for several decades. In his book *Bowling Alone*, he observed an interesting trend in bowlers. In the 1990s, the rate of bowlers in America was at an all time high, and yet few of those bowlers were joining leagues. Putnam hypothesized that a causal relationship exists between the generational decline in social connectedness and depression, suicide, and loneliness.[29] Although Putnam uses bowling as an intriguing example, the decline in social groups and clubs has been a trend across all institutions.

US church membership remained at more than 70% between 1937 and 1976. In the past 2 decades, church membership has decreased by approximately 20% points, with millennial church membership at 42%.[28] Youth sports participation has decreased to 38% in the past decade.[30] Between 1975 and 1999, the average number of times Americans entertained guests in their home decreased by 50%.[29] Membership in the Boy Scouts of America has decreased by more than 26% since 2010.[31] Despite 1.9 million service members deploying to Iraq and Afghanistan in the past 20 years, membership in the Veterans of Foreign Wars (VFW) has decreased by nearly a million members from its peak in 1992.[32,34] The VFW membership decline has correlated with the passing of World War II and Korean War veterans. The younger generation of veterans seem to be less interested in bingo nights and other community-focused activities traditionally offered through the VFW.

Community is a critical component of mental health. Humans are not meant to live in isolation and belonging, support, and purpose are all strengthened by robust communities and organizations. These organizations allow people to engage with like-minded individuals who share similar interests, values, and beliefs. Throughout history, societal needs have changed and organizations have come and gone to address these needs. A decrease in traditional membership organizations may not mean the looming end of civil society, but it may represent an evolution that is occurring in response to the digital and more individualized culture. As individuals reject bowling leagues and bingo nights in favor of Netflix and Instagram, civil society needs to change to respond to new community needs.

TWENTY-FIRST CENTURY PROBLEMS: SOCIAL MEDIA

The explosion of social media seems to provide opportunities to reverse the decrease in social capital. People can seek and find like-minded individuals across the globe, promising an era of connectedness that was unimaginable even 30 years ago. The broad adoption of social media platforms has not reversed the concerning trends; rather, the widespread use of social media seems to correlate with the acceleration of loneliness and declines in social participation. Instead of fostering a small number of deep friendships, social media encourages "friending" hundreds or thousands of people. Friending involves a simple button click and there is no long-term investment into the relationship along with the loss of other traditional traits of close friendship.

Social media has facilitated more engagement in controversial conversations. Historically, one would not discuss religion or politics with a boss or old high school classmate, but these discussions occur frequently online and can lead to the destruction of friendships. Social media has also impacted real-world friendships. Catching up on life events is no longer needed because everyone maintains instant updates through each other's social platforms. The impact of social media on mental health remains uncertain. Many studies have suggested that social media drives negative social comparison and leads to more mental health concerns. Other studies have concluded that social media allows authentic self-presentation and connection with like-minded people regardless of geography, leading to positive user well-being.[35] The lack of consensus in research suggests that the mental health impact of social media is influenced by how individuals use these technologies with underlying strengths or weaknesses in social constructs being accentuated by these platforms.

Technology and social media has provided an imperfect solution to the COVID-19 lockdowns and self-isolation. Video chat platforms have replaced in-person meetings and provide some sense of connection. Elderly adults who may struggle with the uptake of new technology have been at particular risk. Research at the University of Chicago found that the COVID-19 pandemic has resulted in one-third of seniors reporting more loneliness than usual.[36] Studies conducted before the COVID-19 pandemic suggested that senior citizens can combat loneliness with greater adoption of social media and other virtual technology.[37] However, some people report that social media has exacerbated loneliness by serving as a painful reminder of their separation from friends and family. In a recent survey on COVID-19–related loneliness, 10% of respondents indicated that video chats worsened their loneliness.[27]

TWENTY-FIRST CENTURY SOLUTIONS: PSYCHOPHARMACOLOGY

Just as society is undergoing a transformational evolution, psychiatry continues to evolve as well. 50 years ago, the cornerstone of psychiatric care was psychoanalysis and its explanation of mental illness. Although psychotherapy remains an important and critical function of mental health treatment, psychopharmacology has supplanted the psychodynamic approach in the treatment of serious mental illness and continues to expand its role in the treatment of depression, anxiety, and other psychiatric disorders.[38] On the forefront of research, rapid-acting antidepressants show promise in the treatment of severe depression and suicidal urges. Novel antidepressant mechanisms of action including ketamine, neurohormone modulation, nitrous oxide, and hallucinogens provide potential opportunities to change how clinicians treat and manage depressive illness.[39]

Advances in psychopharmacology can improve access to care. Primary care clinicians may not be comfortable prescribing a monoamine oxidase inhibitor or a tricyclic antidepressant owing to serious side effects and drug interactions, but primary care clinicians now readily prescribe selective serotonin reuptake inhibitors owing to their ease of dosing and patient tolerability. Primary care providers account for 79% of antidepressant prescriptions and treat 60% of people diagnosed with depression.[40] This shift in the management of depression and other psychiatric conditions allows psychiatrists and other mental health specialists to see patients with more complex conditions, thus improving access for patients with both mild and severe mental illnesses. Moving forward, primary care providers should continue to embrace their expanded role in treating mental illness and further engage in continuing education for mental health to stay up to date on a rapidly evolving psychopharmacologic landscape.

Although these pharmacologic advancements have led to the greater adoption of medication-oriented treatments for mental illness, this advance does not supplant psychotherapy as an important treatment. Psychotherapy remains a highly effective treatment for many psychiatric disorders. Although there is unsettled debate whether a certain therapeutic approach leads to superior outcomes, meta-analyses consistently endorse psychotherapy as an effective treatment of depression, anxiety, and other conditions.[41,42] As with any illness, mental health conditions require a holistic and comprehensive treatment approach, with clinicians weighing the potential benefits against side effects, cost, tolerability, and compliance. Many patients will benefit from a combination approach of pharmacologic intervention, psychotherapy, lifestyle modification, and psychosocial interventions.

TWENTY-FIRST CENTURY SOLUTIONS: COMMUNITY

The field of behavioral health has historically recognized the importance of psychosocial health. Relationships, family dynamics, employment, education, recreation, and physical health can all impact a patient's emotional well-being. In recent years, psychiatry has moved toward a more integrative approach to treating mental illness. Therapies that were once on the fringe of Western medicine are now frequently covered by insurers. Mindfulness-based interventions have demonstrated efficacy in the treatment of depression, pain, addiction, and other conditions.[43] Light therapy is frequently used to treat seasonal depression with emerging evidence that this intervention may help other psychiatric conditions such as bipolar disorder.[44] A recent review of 1.2 million adults found that regular exercise improves mental health, decreasing the mental health burden by 43%.[45]

Social determinants of health play an outsized role in mental illness. Social determinants of mental health include but are not limited to discrimination, adverse childhood experiences, education, unemployment, income inequality, access to healthy food, housing quality and safety, and community cohesion. Just as a clinician carefully weighs medication options, equal time and energy should be spent to help patients improve the environmental and psychosocial influences of their mental health.[46] The recognition of these social determinants of health has led to further research funding and changes to public health policy. Although local, state, and federal governments enact policy, individual clinicians and practices can make a difference through trauma-informed care, assertive community treatment, and the integration of community programs such as vocational rehabilitation.[47] **Table 1** outlines some common contributing factors to mental health and brief strategies for clinicians to help enact change.

Table 1
Integrative mental health care

Mental Health Factor	How Can Clinicians Help?	Community Referrals
Poor diet/food access	Ask patients about their diets, access to healthy foods, ability to shop at grocery stores	Government programs (SNAP, WIC, Free and reduced school meals, senior meal programs) Nutritional counseling Handouts outlining healthy dietary choices
Exercise/access to exercise (parks, gyms, safe neighborhoods to walk)	Ask patients about specific exercise habits (type of exercise, frequency, level of exertion) Encourage exercise, even small amounts can help, celebrate little victories Educate patients on types of exercise	Gym memberships (reduced rates through insurance or community gym) Physical therapy referral for exercise education Find exercise groups in the area (yoga in the park, walking clubs, etc.)
Stress/external stressors	Assess coping strategies and encourage self-care Teach mindfulness based stress reduction exercises	Referrals for yoga, psychotherapy, engagement in relaxing and enjoyable self-care activities
Poor sleep	Rule out organic causes Inquire and educate on sleep hygiene Consider light therapy	Cognitive–behavioral therapy–Insomnia therapist Community referrals to improve identified lifestyle or sleep hygiene influences
Isolation/stigma	Ask about family, friends, and social supports Ask if patient is comfortable confiding in people around them Educate on mental health/ stigma	Refer to mental health support groups Psychotherapy Online support groups/ Facebook mental health groups
Unemployment/job dissatisfaction	Supportive psychotherapy Coping strategies for stress, mindfulness Identify barriers to employment	Vocational rehabilitation Job coaching School (often grants for mental health available)

TWENTY-FIRST CENTURY SOLUTIONS: TECHNOLOGY

Technological advancement has led to new social problems, but also has created opportunities to improve health care delivery and outcomes. Telemedicine was already one of the fastest growing sectors of health care and the COVID-19 pandemic has accelerated its widespread adoption and acceptance. Telepsychiatry is the delivery of mental health care remotely through the implementation of technology. Telepsychiatry encompasses video chat, telephone communication, and other forms of technological communication including text and email. Telepsychiatry can improve the patient care experience, improve population health, decrease costs, and improve the provider experience.[48] Virtual visits allow increased access to care because access is not limited to patient or provider location. Cost is also decreased because patients and providers do not spend time and money commuting, with care delivered in a discrete and comfortable environment.[49,50]

The investments made into telemedicine in response to COVID-19 will likely change the role of telemedicine in the postpandemic health care landscape. Patients may use telehealth as a form of "forward triage," preempting unnecessary sick visits to the primary care office, urgent care, or emergency department.[51] This form of health care triage can provide opportunities for cost savings across all medical specialties. One of the barriers to the permanent adoption of telepsychiatry will be payer reimbursement. Policy must be changed at the state and federal levels to cement telemedicine as a permanent fixture of the health care delivery model.

Telemedicine offers opportunities to change the way patients access mental health care. The Centers for Medicare and Medicaid Services now authorizes payment for behavioral health integration services. These changes now allow a psychiatric medical professional to contract with primary care offices to provide consultations. The primary care office uses validated rating scales to identify patients who are struggling with mental health issues. Once identified, the consulting psychiatric provider provides prescribing guidance and treatment recommendations.[52] This innovative approach of care integration expands the reach of psychiatric prescribers who are in increasingly short supply, allows for mental health care in rural areas that may not have psychiatric services, and improves the identification of mental health issues because patients are screened proactively in the primary care setting.

A driving force behind the telemedicine revolution is the broad access to home or mobile internet. Compared with 2011, American smartphone ownership has increased from 35% to 81%.[53] Most US adults now possess the ability to video conference with their medical provider. The prevalence of smartphones also provides a window into the future of psychiatric diagnosis and treatment. Mobile phone apps that target mental health have flooded the marketplace. A 2017 report found 490 unique apps designed for mental health disorders.[54] Apps provide the potential to reduce the barriers of affordability, access, stigma, and time constraints. Research regarding mental health app efficacy is limited, but does show promise.[55–59] The importance of mobile apps and wearable technology such as smart watches will continue to grow as technology advances.

Researchers are working on strategies to incorporate artificial intelligence into psychiatry, often through mobile applications. Companies like IBM are developing programs that analyze speech to identify early indicators of developmental disorders, neurodegenerative conditions, and mental health decompensation.[60,61] Machine learning can also be used in passive applications that monitor behavior through smart device use to identify trends that suggest mental health changes, such as increased screen time, decreased physical activity, or search word clusters.[62] Current technology does not threaten to replace clinicians with machine learning algorithms. Previous research has shown that some psychiatrist's placebo worked better than others, suggesting that personal connection and therapeutic alliance plays a key role in treatment success.[63] A book overviewing the efficacy of therapy argued that the therapist plays a greater role in outcomes than therapeutic technique, theory, or structure.[64] In the near future, mobile applications and artificial intelligence may fully incorporate into clinical practice and serve as tools for diagnostic clarity and outcomes tracking. This technology promises to improve access and outcomes for patients and should be welcomed and embraced by clinicians.

SUMMARY

Medicine has always been tied to cultural norms and beliefs. Perceptions of health, disease prevention, and how people seek help are concepts that have evolved in response to cultural changes and needs throughout the years. Mental health care has evolved from an outlier of medicine that relied on created terminology to describe poorly understood phenomena, to a rapidly evolving specialty that offers biologic underpinnings for ailments and conditions. Changes in cultural norms also lead to shifts in causes and contributing factors of mental health. Western society has become more individualized and the shift away from community involvement requires a change in how clinicians assess and treat mental illness.

As a society, adaptation to cultural disruption has occurred before. Although the Industrial Revolution led to social and economic disruption, many organizations were formed in response to the urban migration of the nineteenth century that remain bedrocks of current civil society. Before urbanization, charity was administered by families, churches, and members of the small town community. Nonprofit organizations such The United Way, Salvation Army, and YMCA were created in response to a new societal need. The digital revolution promises to be as equally disruptive as the Industrial Revolution 2 centuries ago. The COVID-19 crisis will likely accelerate societal transformation as well. After centuries of urbanization, will people begin to shift back to rural towns as they become untethered from the need to work in an office or factory? Medical providers must take their role seriously as front-line soldiers in the battle against loneliness and other mental health struggles that may develop in response to economic disruption and cultural change.

Clinicians of the future should embrace an integrative approach to mental health. Helping patients to find new housing, a new job, or teaching about exercise are all interventions that can provide impactful improvement in mental health and outcomes. Incorporating technology including telemedicine, mobile applications, and alternative care delivery models are all innovations that can help the health care system adapt to the changing needs of an evolving society. Although change brings new challenges, necessity is the mother of invention. The future of mental health care is bright and the profession is ready to tackle new problems thoughtfully, respectfully, and patient-focused.

DISCLOSURE

M. Asbach is a paid speaker/consultant for Abbvie Pharmaceuticals, Neurocrine Biosciences, Otsuka Pharmaceutical, Avanir Pharmaceuticals. The author has no conflicts of interest to report and received no funding for this article.

REFERENCES

1. Porter R. Madness: a brief history. New York: Oxford University Press; 2002.

2. Millon T. Masters of the mind: exploring the story of mental illness from anxiety times to the new millennium. Hoboken (NJ): Wiley; 2004.
3. Evans KM. "Interrupted by fits of weeping": Cicero's major depressive disorder and the death of Tullia. Hist Psychiatry 2007;18(1):81–102.
4. Anderson RD. The history of witchcraft: a review with some psychiatric comments. Am J Psychiatry 1970;126(12):1727–35.
5. Elder R, Evans K, Nizette D. Psychiatric & mental health nursing. Mosby Australia: Elsevier; 2008.
6. Sasse B. Them. New York: St Martins Press; 2018.
7. Occupational Employment Statistics. U.S. Bureau of Labor Statistics. Available at: https://www.bls.gov/oes/current/area_emp_chart/area_emp_chart.htm. Accessed June 27, 2020.
8. Manyika J, Lund S, Chui M, et al. Jobs lost, jobs gained: what the future of work will mean for jobs, skills, and wages. McKinsey & Company; 2017. Available at: https://www.mckinsey.com/featured-insights/future-of-work/jobs-lost-jobs-gained-what-the-future-of-work-will-mean-for-jobs-skills-and-wages#. Accessed June 27, 2020.
9. Killc K, Marin D. How COVID-19 is transforming the world economy. VOX CEPR Policy Portal. 2020. Available at: https://voxeu.org/article/how-covid-19-transforming-world-economy. Accessed June 27, 2020.
10. Vilhelmson B, Thulin E. Who and where are the flexible workers? Exploring the current diffusion of telework in Sweden. New Technol Work Employ 2016;31(1). https://doi.org/10.1111/ntwe.12060.
11. Vries HD, Tummers L, Bekkers V. The benefits of teleworking in the public sector: reality or rhetoric? Rev Public Pers Adm 2019;39(4):570–93.
12. Batic-Mujanovic O, Poric S, Pranjic N, et al. Influence of unemployment on mental health of the working age population. Mater Sociomed 2017;29(2):92–6.
13. Ng KH, Agius M, Zaman R. The global economic crisis: effects on mental health and what can be done. J R Soc Med 2013;106(6):211–4.
14. Eisenberg P, Lazarsfeld PF. The psychological effects of unemployment. Psychol Bull 1938;35:358–90.
15. Butterworth P, Leach LS, Strazdins L, et al. The psychosocial quality of work determines whether employment has benefits for mental health: results from a longitudinal national household panel survey. Occup Environ Med 2011;68(11):806–12.
16. Moody L, Satterwhite E, Bickel WK. Substance use in rural central Appalachia: current status and treatment considerations. Rural Ment Health 2017;41(2):123–35.
17. Schreuder C. The 1995 Chicago heat wave. Chicago Tribune; , 2015. Available at: https://www.chicagotribune.com/nation-world/chi-chicagodays-1995heat-story-story.html. Accessed June 19, 2020.
18. Klinenberg E. Dying alone: an interview with Erik Klineberg. Chicago IL: University of Chicago Press; 2002. Available at: https://press.uchicago.edu/Misc/Chicago/443213in.html. Accessed June 19, 2020.
19. Holt-Lunstad J, Smith TB, Baker M, et al. Loneliness and social isolation as risk factors for mortality: a meta-analytic review. Perspect Psychol Sci 2015;10(2):227–37.
20. The "Loneliness Epidemic." U.S. Health and Resources & Services Administration. 2019. Available at: https://www.hrsa.gov/enews/past-issues/2019/january-17/loneliness-epidemic. Accessed June 19, 2020.
21. Rico-Uribe LA, Caballero FF, Martín-María N, et al. Association of loneliness with all-cause mortality: a meta-analysis. PLoS One 2018;13(1):e0190033.

22. Case A, Deaton A. Rising morbidity and mortality in midlife among white non-Hispanic Americans in the 21st century. Proc Natl Acad Sci U S A 2015; 112(49):15078–83.

23. National Marriage and Divorce Rates. Centers for Disease Control and Prevention. Available at: https://www.cdc.gov/nchs/data/dvs/national-marriage-divorce-rates-00-18.pdf. Accessed June 19, 2020.

24. Hurst G. All the lonely people...are men: a fifth have no friends. The Times UK. Available at: https://www.thetimes.co.uk/article/all-the-lonely-people-are-men-a-fifth-have-no-friends-6rzvhl736?region=global. Accessed June 19, 2020.

25. Klinenberg E. Heat wave: a social autopsy of disaster in Chicago. Chicago, IL: University of Chicago Press; 2002.

26. Report: loneliness and anxiety during lockdown. SocialPro. 2020. Available at: https://socialpronow.com/loneliness-corona/. . Accessed June 20, 2020.

27. Price S. Nearly half of Americans are struggling with loneliness amid social distancing and many don't know where to find help. ValuePenguin. 2020. Available at: https://www.valuepenguin.com/coronavirus-loneliness-survey?utm_source=STAT+Newsletters&utm_campaign=f3e6bb82c2-MR_COPY_01&utm_medium=email&utm_term=0_8cab1d7961-f3e6bb82c2-152047705. Accessed June 20, 2020.

28. Loneliness is at epidemic levels in America. Cigna. 2020. Available at: https://www.cigna.com/about-us/newsroom/studies-and-reports/combatting-loneliness/. Accessed June 10, 2020.

29. Putnam RD. Bowling alone: the collapse and revival of American community. New York: Simon and Schuster; 2000.

30. Survey: kids quit most sports by age 11. The Aspen Institute Project Play. 2019. Available at: https://www.aspenprojectplay.org/national-youth-sport-survey/1. Accessed June 20, 2020.

31. Schmidt S, Epstein K. Lawsuits. Possible bankruptcy. Declining numbers. Is there a future for the Boy Scouts? The Washington Post. 2019. Available at: https://www.washingtonpost.com/local/social-issues/lawsuits-possible-bankruptcy-declining-members-is-there-a-future-for-the-boy-scouts/2019/09/11/54699d6a-ce53-11e9-8c1c-7c8ee785b855_story.html. Accessed June 19, 2020.

32. Institute of Medicine (US). Committee on the initial Assessment of Readjustment needs of Military Personnel, veterans, and their families. Returning home from Iraq and Afghanistan: preliminary assessment of readjustment needs of veterans, service members, and their families. Washington (DC): National Academies Press (US); 2010.

33. Operation enduring freedom and Operation Iraqi Freedom: demographics and impact. Available at: https://www.ncbi.nlm.nih.gov/books/NBK220068/. Accessed June 20,2020.

34. VFW snaps 27 year membership decline. Veteran of Foreign Wars. 2019. Available at: https://www.vfw.org/media-and-events/latest-releases/archives/2019/7/vfw-snaps-27-year-membership-decline. Accessed June 20, 2020.

35. Berryman C, Ferguson CJ, Negy C. Social media use and mental health among young adults. Psychiatr Q 2018;89:307–14.

36. More than half of older adults already experiencing disruptions in care as a result of coronavirus. NORC at the University of Chicago. Interview Dates April 10-15, 2020. Available at: https://www.norc.org/PDFs/JAHF%20TSF/JAHF_TSF_NORC_topline_42720.pdf. Accessed June 28, 2020.

37. Ducharme J. COVID-19 is making America's loneliness epidemic even worse. TIME. 2020. Available at: https://time.com/5833681/loneliness-covid-19/. Accessed June 27,2020.
38. Nasrallah H. From bedlam to biomarkers: the transformation of psychiatry's terminology reflects its 4 conceptual earthquakes. Curr Psychtr 2015;14(1):5–7.
39. Nasrallah H. Transformative advances are unfolding in psychiatry. Curr Psychtr 2019;18(9):10–2.
40. Barkil-Oteo A. Collaborative care for depression in primary care: how psychiatry could "troubleshoot" current treatments and practices. Yale J Biol Med 2013; 86(2):139–46. Available at: https://www.ncbi.nlm.nih.gov/pmc/articles/PMC3670434/. Accessed June 27, 2020.
41. Cuijpers P, Van Straten A, Andersson G, et al. Psychotherapy for depression in adults: a meta-analysis of comparative outcome studies. J Consult Clin Psychol 2008;76(6):909–22.
42. Cuijpers P, Sijbrandij M, Koole SL, et al. The efficacy of psychotherapy and pharmacotherapy in treating depressive and anxiety disorders: a meta-analysis of direct comparisons. World Psychiatry 2013;12(2):137–48.
43. Goldberg SB, Tucker RP, Greene PA, et al. Mindfulness-based interventions for psychiatric disorders: a systematic review and meta-analysis. Clin Psychol Rev 2018;59:52–60.
44. Sit DK, McGowan J, Wiltrout C, et al. Adjunctive bright light therapy for bipolar depression: a randomized double-blind placebo-controlled trial. Am J Psychiatry 2017;175(2):131–9.
45. Chekroud SR, Gueorguieva R, Zheutlin AB, et al. Association between physical exercise and mental health in 1·2 million individuals in the USA between 2011 and 2015: a cross-sectional study. Lancet Psychiatry 2018;5(9):739–46.
46. Compton MT, Shim RS. The social determinants of mental health. Clin Synth 2015. https://doi.org/10.1176/appi.focus.20150017.
47. Shim RS, Compton MT. Addressing the social determinants of mental health: if not now, when? if not us, who? Psychiatr Serv 2018;69(8):844–6.
48. Shore J. The evolution and history of telepsychiatry and its impact on psychiatric care: current implications for psychiatrists and psychiatric organizations. Int Rev Psychiatry 2015;27:469–75.
49. Chakrabarti S. Usefulness of telepsychiatry: a critical evaluation of videoconferencing-based approaches. World J Psychiatry 2015;5:286–304.
50. Deslich S, Stec B, Tomblin S, et al. Telepsychiatry in the 21st century: transforming healthcare with technology. Perspect Health Inf Manag 2013;10.
51. Hollander JE, Carr BG. Virtually Perfect? Telemedicine for Covid-19. N Engl J Med 2020;382(18):1679–81.
52. Behavioral Health Integration Services. MLN booklet. centers for Medicare & Medicaid Services. Available at: https://www.cms.gov/Outreach-and-Education/Medicare-Learning-Network-MLN/MLNProducts/Downloads/BehavioralHealthIntegration.pdf. Accessed June 27,2020.
53. Internet & Technology. Mobile fact sheet. Pew research center. June 12 2019. Available at: https://www.pewresearch.org/internet/fact-sheet/mobile/. Accessed June 27, 2020.
54. Aitkin M, Clancy B, Nass D. The growing value of digital health. IQVIA Institute for Human Data Science; 2017. Available at: https://www.iqvia.com/insights/the-iqvia-institute/reports/the-growing-value-of-digital-health. Accessed June 27, 2020.

55. Twomey C, O'Reilly G, Meyer B. Effectiveness of an individually-tailored compu-terised CBT programme (Deprexis) for depression: a meta-analysis. Psychiatry Res 2017;256:371–7.
56. Huguet A, Rao S, McGrath PJ, et al. A systematic review of cognitive behavioral therapy and behavioral activation apps for depression. PLoS One 2016;11(5): e0154248.
57. Wright JH, Owen JJ, Richards D, et al. Computer-assisted cognitive-behavior therapy for depression: a systematic review and meta-analysis. J Clin Psychiatry 2019;80(2):18r12188.
58. Kerst A, Zielasek J, Gaebel W. Smartphone applications for depression: a sys-tematic literature review and a survey of health care professionals' attitudes to-wards their use in clinical practice. Eur Arch Psychiatry Clin Neurosci 2020; 270(2):139–52.
59. Weisel KK, Fuhrmann LM, Berking M, et al. Standalone smartphone apps for mental health-a systematic review and meta-analysis. NPJ Digit Med 2019;2:118.
60. With AI. our words will be a window into our mental health. IBM. Available at: https://www.research.ibm.com/5-in-5/mental-health/. Accessed June 27, 2020.
61. Ben-Zeev D, Wang R, Abdullah S, et al. Mobile behavioral sensing for outpatients and inpatients with schizophrenia. Psychiatr Serv 2016;67(5):558–61.
62. Wang R, Aung MSH, Abdullah S, et al. CrossCheck: toward passive sensing and detection of mental health changes in people with schizophrenia. UBICOMP '16. Available at: https://dl.acm.org/doi/pdf/10.1145/2971648.2971740. Accessed June 27, 2020.
63. McKay KM, Imel ZE, Wampold BE. Psychiatrist effects in the psychopharmaco-logical treatment of depression. J Affect Disord 2006;92(2–3):287–90.
64. Wampold B, Imel Z. The great psychotherapy debate. New York: Routledge; 2015. https://doi.org/10.4324/9780203582015. Available at:.

Moving?

Make sure your subscription moves with you!

To notify us of your new address, find your **Clinics Account Number** (located on your mailing label above your name), and contact customer service at:

Email: journalscustomerservice-usa@@elsevier.com

800-654-2452 (subscribers in the U.S. & Canada)
314-447-8871 (subscribers outside of the U.S. & Canada)

Fax number: 314-447-8029

Elsevier Health Sciences Division
Subscription Customer Service
3251 Riverport Lane
Maryland Heights, MO 63043

*To ensure uninterrupted delivery of your subscription,
please notify us at least 4 weeks in advance of move.

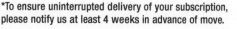

ELSEVIER

Moving?

Make sure your subscription moves with you!

To notify us of your new address, find your Clinics Account Number (located on your mailing label above your name), and contact customer service at:

Email: journalscustomerservice-usa@elsevier.com

800-654-2452 (subscribers in the U.S. & Canada)
314-447-8871 (subscribers outside of the U.S. & Canada)

Fax number: 314-447-8029

Elsevier Health Sciences Division
Subscription Customer Service
3251 Riverport Lane
Maryland Heights, MO 63043